Understanding
Allergies

Dr Joanne Clough

Published by Family Doctor Publications Limited
in association with the British Medical Association

© Family Doctor Publications 2002–2005
Updated 2004, 2005

Family Doctor Publications, PO Box 4664, Poole, Dorset BH15 1NN

ISBN: 1 903474 18 3

Contents

About the author

 Dr Joanne Clough trained at University College Hospital, London, spent two years as an MRC Research Fellow in Australia, and is currently Senior Lecturer in Paediatric Medicine at the University of Southampton and Honorary Consultant Paediatrician at Southampton University Hospital.

Introduction

What is allergy?
Allergy results from an over-reaction of the immune system to a substance that is normally harmless. Many different parts of the body may be affected.

Allergy in modern society
The number of people in the United Kingdom with allergies has increased threefold over the last 20 years and continues to rise. One in three of the UK population now suffers from a medical problem caused by or associated with allergy, a total of 18 million people. It is predicted that a similar increase will be seen in developing countries as they become more westernised.

Many of the factors thought to be responsible for the increase in allergic diseases are related to our western lifestyle. These include our unnaturally refined diet, the early introduction of certain foods to the infant diet, our style of housing, the popularity of indoor furry pets, the increased exposure to chemicals that may cause allergies, the tendency for smaller households with fewer people and our exposure to tobacco smoke.

Many of these factors are especially potent in small children, so it is this age group that is most affected by the rising incidence of allergy.

Allergic disease is the reason for six per cent of all appointments in general practice, and takes up £900 million of the primary care budget. A recent report by the Royal College of Physicians has highlighted that allergic disease in the UK has become not just more common, but also more severe and more complex.

However, there are insufficient specialist allergy centres in the UK, and most GPs have had no clinical training in allergy. Currently, there is only one consultant allergist for every two million people, whereas in other specialties – for example, cardiology – there is one consultant for every 100,000 people.

The Royal College of Physicians is trying to address this problem and many more allergy specialists are in training. In the meantime, better patient education is vital. The more that you can learn about your allergies, the better equipped you will be to manage the problems presented by them in everyday life.

Allergic diseases are chronic in nature, that is, they are persistent, recurring over many months or years. People with allergies don't necessarily look ill, but they are not perfectly well either. Having an allergy problem can interfere with your sleep, making you tired, and may affect your appetite and decrease your ability to concentrate.

All these add up to make you feel less than 100 per cent, and in the long term both your family life and your time at school or work may suffer.

As the symptoms of allergic disease often increase slowly over time, you may not realise how big an impact they are having on your life. Low-level symptoms such as coughing, sneezing or sniffing are accepted as 'normal', and you may end up with lower expectations of what you can manage.

The role of allergies in common diseases

The most common diseases in which allergy plays a part are asthma, hay fever (also called allergic rhinitis), allergies affecting the skin (including eczema and contact dermatitis) and food allergy.

Allergy and asthma

Asthma causes episodes of wheezing, coughing and shortness of breath that can be triggered by a range of things, including the common cold, exercise, contact with furry animals, a high pollen count and exposure to tobacco smoke.

It is a frequent problem in children, affecting as many as one in seven school-aged children. Asthma is slightly less common in adults – affecting about one in ten – but is still a major cause of ill-health. Although many studies have confirmed that asthma is becoming more common, little is known about why.

Allergy and hay fever

Hay fever may be a seasonal condition, causing symptoms in late spring and summer, or may be perennial, causing problems all year round. Its symptoms might not sound serious – a running or blocked nose, watery itchy eyes and sneezing – but they make the lives of hay fever sufferers a misery, and interfere with work, study and sleep.

The exact number of people with hay fever is difficult to judge, but it is thought that as many as 20 per cent of the British population have hay fever at some stage in their lives.

Skin allergy

Skin allergies may take several different forms.

Probably the best known is eczema, but other problems such as contact dermatitis, urticaria (hives) and facial swelling (angio-oedema) may also result from an allergy. Although skin allergy can affect both sexes, more women in particular are developing new allergies. This may be because the average woman uses five different cosmetic and skin care products on her skin every day, and these are likely to contain around 100 different chemicals, any one of which could cause an allergic reaction.

Food allergy

Unpleasant reactions to food are common, but not all of them are caused by allergy. Although almost a fifth of people in the UK think that they are allergic to at least one food, the actual figure is much lower – about two per cent.

Allergy is often incorrectly blamed for causing symptoms that are not truly allergic in nature, because there are a number of other reasons why a food might disagree with you, including food intolerance, a sensitivity to food and food aversion.

Misdiagnosis of allergy

The problem of misdiagnosis is not confined to food allergy. Allergy seems to have become fashionable, particularly among young women. In addition, some alternative practitioners use tests that have not been scientifically assessed and these tests may incorrectly diagnose allergy.

The careful and accurate diagnosis of allergic problems is important for two reasons. First, sufferers may make major changes in their diet or in their lifestyle, in the belief that they have an allergic disease, and these changes may interfere with the quality of their lives for no good reason because they will not cure the problem. Second, labelling their condition incorrectly prevents them from discovering the true reason for their problem and then finding the best treatment for it.

This book explains what happens in the body when an allergy occurs and how to discover whether or not allergy is the cause of your problem. It also describes the different ways of diagnosing allergy and discusses the different treatments available. Finally, useful information about living with allergies is given.

If you have an allergy-related condition, this book should help you to find your way through the maze of diagnosis and treatment. No book can be a substitute for consultation with a doctor, but by making you better informed and well prepared, this book will help you to be more in control of your allergic problems and so to manage them better.

KEY POINTS

- Allergy is becoming more common

- One in three people in the UK is affected by allergy

- Allergy is often misdiagnosed

- There are too few specialist allergy clinics in the UK

What is allergy?

The body's defence system

The human body has a sophisticated defence system that has evolved to protect us against a range of threats, including micro-organisms (such as bacteria, viruses and parasites), chemical substances and even cancer.

This defence system, the immune system, is made up of a large number of different cell types and special proteins. These work together in a complex way to enable us to distinguish our own normal cells ('self') from harmful cells ('non-self') and so to destroy abnormal or invading cells. However, occasionally the immune system reacts to substances that are harmless.

An allergic reaction is an overreaction of the immune defence system to a normally harmless environmental substance. The resulting allergic reaction causes damage to the surrounding tissues, leading to troublesome or even life-threatening consequences.

The term 'allergy' is sometimes used to describe just about any kind of illness. In this book, the term is used much more precisely to mean an exaggerated and inappropriate response of the immune system to a substance that is normally harmless.

An allergic reaction involves different parts of the immune system, including the white blood cells, the spleen, the lymph nodes, the thymus gland and the many small glands within the lining of the respiratory and intestinal tracts.

There are several different types of white blood cells, including lymphocytes, neutrophils, eosinophils, mast cells and macrophages. All of these are controlled by hormones (chemical messengers that trigger specific effects in the body).

In the healthy person

The prime purpose of the immune system is to protect us from micro-organisms that might otherwise kill us. When one of these, such as the measles virus or the bacterium *Staphylococcus aureus*, attacks the body for the first time, cells called macrophages within the lymph nodes, lungs or bowel recognise it as foreign (non-self) because of certain protein molecules, known as antigens, on its surface, and these cells bring it to the attention of the lymphocytes (white blood cells).

One type of lymphocyte, the T lymphocyte, produces protein messengers that stimulate other cells (the B lymphocytes) to produce purpose-built proteins called antibodies. These antibodies are specifically made to fit with and bind onto the antigens on the invading cell's surface. Once there, they send signals to teams of killer cells, which move in and kill the invader.

Each time a different antigen is met, antibodies are made specifically against it, and the body can make millions of different ones. The process of recognising an antigen and making antibodies against it for the first time is called sensitisation.

It may take a few days for the body's response to reach full strength. However, for the rest of your life your immune system is able to remember each harmful

How the immune system deals with harmful cells

The immune (defence) system is made up of many different cell types that work together to enable the body to distinguish between its own cells ('self') and harmful cells ('non-self'). The following sequence of five illustrations is a representation of how the immune system works to destroy invading micro-organisms.

Broken skin

Invading bacterium

Blood vessel

1. Bacteria invade the body through broken skin. The damaged tissues release chemicals that attract white blood cells called macrophages

Macrophages destroying invading cells

Porous blood vessel

2. These chemicals also cause the underlying blood vessels to dilate, increasing the blood supply to the area and making the vessels more leaky, which causes the characteristics of inflammation and also allows macrophages to reach the invading cells

How the immune system deals with harmful cells (contd)

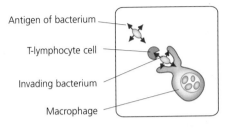

Antigen of bacterium

T-lymphocyte cell

Invading bacterium

Macrophage

3. Some of the invading cells are destroyed by being engulfed by macrophages. T lymphocytes send signals to B lymphocytes to make specific antibodies to deal with the invader

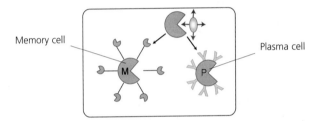

Memory cell

Plasma cell

4. The T lymphocyte stimulates the production of two types of B lymphocyte: plasma cells which produce antibodies for immediate use and memory cells which are stored for future use

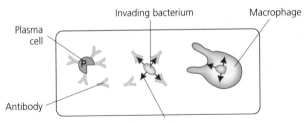

Invading bacterium

Macrophage

Plasma cell

Antibody

Antigen of bacterium

5. If the body is again threatened by the same bacteria, T lymphocytes stimulate the plasma cells to produce antibodies which bind onto the matching antigens on the invading cell's surface. The antibodies then send signals to 'killer' cells called macrophages that move in and destroy the invader

micro-organism and, if the same organism attacks again, it is immediately recognised. No other organ of the body apart from the brain has the property of memory.

If the same micro-organism strikes again, as soon as its unique antigens are recognised, the T lymphocytes send chemical messages to the group of B lymphocytes that have a specific memory for that invader.

These multiply very quickly and produce large quantities of antibody, which helps to kill the harmful organisms. Other white cells produce chemicals such as histamine, which increases the blood supply to the area involved and makes the blood vessels more leaky. This allows other helpful white blood cell types, such as the macrophage, which are able to eat and destroy the invading cells, to reach the area.

We can see evidence of the effects of histamine when a skin wound becomes infected. The area becomes red and swollen because of the increased blood supply, and may be hot and sore as a result of the chemicals produced in the course of the immune reaction. This process is known as inflammation.

In the allergic person

When you develop an allergy, your immune system still works perfectly well against the antigens associated with viruses, bacteria and parasites, but, in addition, it also reacts to other antigens that should be completely harmless.

These antigens are known as allergens. These are incorrectly seen as being dangerous by your immune system, which mounts an immune response against them. This response is called an allergic reaction, and you will have developed an allergy.

Sensitisation

There are two stages in the development of an allergy, and the first is sensitisation (see page 7 and figure on page 12). This process happens when an allergen is encountered by the immune system and antibodies are made against it, despite it being harmless.

These are a special type of antibody, known as immunoglobulin E or IgE for short – immunoglobulin is another name for an antibody. They are of the same type as those that protect us against parasites such as worms, flukes and amoebae.

Parasites are much larger than other micro-organisms such as viruses and bacteria, and the body has had to find alternative ways of getting rid of them. IgE is different from other types of antibody in that it can attach itself on to special cells called mast cells and basophils, which contain thousands of toxic granules. These toxic granules are released when an allergen binds to the IgE on the cell surface, causing the symptoms that we associate with allergy.

You do not always become sensitised the first time that your body meets a particular allergen – a substance may be tolerated for many years before an allergy develops. Sensitisation does not produce any symptoms and you will not be aware that it is happening. After sensitisation, the immune system retains a memory of the allergen and will recognise it if it meets it again.

Allergic reactions

Once you have been sensitised, even a tiny quantity of that allergen can lead to an allergic reaction. The allergen binds to the IgE present on the surface of the mast cells and basophils, and the toxic granules are released.

How an allergy develops

There are two stages in the development of an allergy: first sensitisation which does not produce any symptoms and then the allergic reaction.

Sensitisation

Sensitisation occurs when your body meets an allergen, recognises it as foreign and your white blood cells make a memory of it.

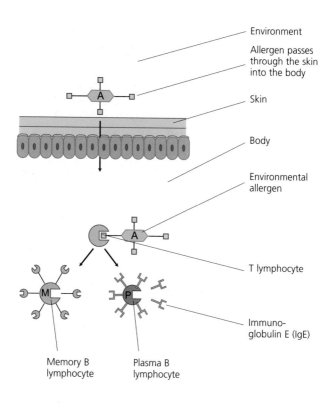

Environment

Allergen passes through the skin into the body

Skin

Body

Environmental allergen

T lymphocyte

Immuno-globulin E (IgE)

Memory B lymphocyte

Plasma B lymphocyte

How an allergy develops (contd)

Allergic reaction

Environment

Allergen passes through the skin into the body

Skin

Body

Allergen

1. Once the body is sensitised, if this allergen is met again, even a tiny amount can produce an allergic reaction

IgE antibody

Memory B lymphocyte

Plasma B lymphocyte

2. The allergen is recognised and this triggers the production of large quantities of the IgE antibody by the memory B lymphocytes

IgE antibody

Mast cell

Toxic granules

3. Some of the IgE antibody attaches to mast cells which contain toxic granules

Allergen

IgE antibody

Toxic chemicals released

Mast cell

4. The allergen causes the severe reaction as IgE links molecules present on the surface of the mast cell. The mast cell bursts releasing toxic chemicals which then cause the symptoms that we associate with allergy

These contain potent irritant chemicals such as histamine and a number of different enzymes. If this reaction were the result of a parasitic infection, these chemicals would help to kill and digest the invading organisms.

If, however, the immune system is reacting against a harmless allergen such as pollen, these substances serve no useful purpose, but instead cause an increase in the blood supply to the tissues, leakage of fluid from the small blood vessels and local irritation. The result is hotness, redness, itching and swelling in the affected area, and the production of excess watery secretions.

In addition, the muscles of the airways in the lungs and the bowel may go into spasm, causing wheezing, shortness of breath, abdominal colic and diarrhoea. This process gives us the symptoms that we associate with allergy.

Once you have developed an allergy, your body will always produce an allergic reaction whenever it meets even minute amounts of this allergen again. However, the reaction will not necessarily be exactly the same each time. A number of things can affect the type and the extent of an allergic reaction. These include the amount or dose of allergen involved, the part of your body exposed to the allergen, whether there are other factors present that enhance your allergic reaction (for example, a high level of air pollutants), and even how unwell you are at the time. In addition, the pattern of your allergic reactions may change as you get older. Some may become less pronounced with age, and it is even possible to 'grow out of' an allergy.

What are the most common allergens?

All allergens are made of proteins – organic compounds made of hydrogen, oxygen and nitrogen that are found in all living organisms. Occasionally, a non-protein substance can act as an allergen (for example, penicillin and other drugs), but only because they can attach themselves to a small protein molecule called a hapten inside the body. Virtually any protein can act as an allergen and new ones are being discovered all the time. The allergens most commonly causing allergies in the UK are described below.

House-dust mites

The house-dust mite is too small to be seen by the naked eye. It loves warm, humid conditions and large numbers can be found inside mattresses, bedding,

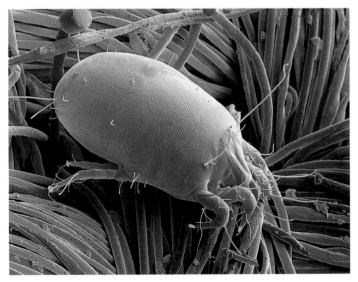

Electron micrograph of a house-dust mite.

pillows, soft furnishings and cuddly toys. House-dust mite allergy has become more common in recent times because double glazing, loft and wall insulation, and other energy-saving measures reduce ventilation inside our houses and encourage the warm, moist conditions that the house-dust mite needs.

The mite lives off scales of human skin which we constantly shed and which make up the majority of house dust. It is not the mites themselves but their faecal particles that act as an allergen and cause allergies. These particles are so small that they can be suspended in the air for long periods of time and so can be inhaled though the nose and into the lungs, where they can cause the symptoms of hay fever and asthma. When they come into direct contact with the skin, they can cause eczema. At least three-quarters of all allergy sufferers in the UK are allergic to the house-dust mite.

Grass and tree pollen

Pollens are the male reproductive part of plants (or trees) that fertilise other plants of the same species. They consist of small grains and are carried to another flower by either insects or the wind. Wind pollination is not very efficient, and so plants that reproduce in this way produce vast quantities of pollen. The airborne pollens are very light and can be carried in the air for long periods of time. When these particles reach the eyes, nose or lungs of a sensitised person, they cause an allergic reaction commonly described as hay fever. If breathed into the lungs they can, in addition, make asthma worse.

Different plants produce their pollens at different times of the year and it is possible, using a pollen

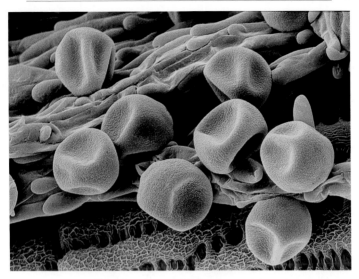
Electron micrograph of pollen grains.

calendar, to work out which plants might be responsible for your symptoms. The most common culprit is grass pollen, which is around from late April to early September.

Animal dander (skin scales and hair)

Most furry animals can cause an allergy as a result of the allergens in their skin scales, hair, urine and saliva. These allergens can be spread widely throughout our homes, not just by animals but also on our clothing and shoes.

Seven out of ten British households have a pet of some kind and pet allergens cause about 40 per cent of all childhood asthma. Allergy to pets does not only occur in their owners. These allergens are so potent and long lasting that they are easily spread, for

Electron micrograph of a human hair on the skin surface.

example by contact with bus seats, to non-pet owners, who can be exposed to enough allergen in their everyday life to become sensitised.

Food allergens

Many foods can act as allergens. The most common in children under the age of five are cows' milk and hens' eggs. Over the age of five years, other allergies are more common – such as to peanuts (which is not a true nut but a legume, that is, it grows as a seed in a pod like a pea), tree nuts, fish and shellfish.

Food allergies can take different forms, ranging from episodes of mild symptoms to life-threatening attacks.

Cows' milk

Hens' eggs

Peanuts

Tree nuts, e.g. walnuts

Shellfish

Fish

Many foods can act as allergens; the most common are shown.

Moulds and spores

The spores from certain moulds and plants can trigger allergic reactions in some people, particularly in the autumn.

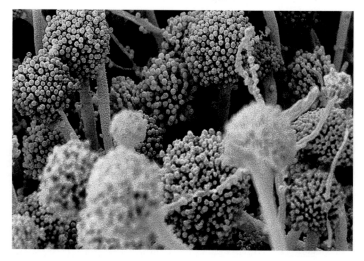

Electron micrograph of the fruiting bodies and spores of the fungus *Rhizopus oligosporus.*

Drug allergies

Certain drugs, particularly some antibiotics, can cause allergic reactions. An allergy will never occur the first time a drug is administered but may do so on any subsequent occasion, even if the drug has been well tolerated in the past.

Insect stings

Although everyone finds insect stings unpleasant, in some people these can trigger severe allergic reactions. Stings by bees and wasps are most commonly responsible.

A common adult worker wasp – *Vespula vulgaris.*

Who develops allergies?
Family history

Although we do not completely understand why it is that some people develop allergies and others do not, it is clear that allergies have a tendency to run in families. This inherited tendency towards allergy is called atopy.

In the near future it is likely that the genes (a gene is a small part of our genetic code made of DNA) responsible for atopy will be identified.

Atopic people produce excess quantities of the allergy antibody (IgE) when they come into contact with substances in their environment that can act as allergens.

Environmental factors

Although atopy is inherited, environmental factors also play a part in the development of allergic disorders. This is why not all members of a family, indeed not even both of a pair of identical twins, are affected to the same extent. Factors operating in early life, probably even during pregnancy, act together with the degree of allergy genes that you inherited from your parents to determine whether or not allergy develops. These early life factors include the timing of your first exposure to the allergen and the size of that exposure – however atopic you are, if you were never exposed to any allergen, you would not develop allergies. The number of viral infections suffered in early childhood may also have an effect – these infections seem to be protective against the development of allergy. High levels of exposure to tobacco smoke in pregnancy and early life increase an individual's risk of becoming atopic.

So a baby, born to cigarette-smoking, cat-owning, atopic parents, whose birth coincides with the pollen season, who spends his or her first months in a well-insulated double-glazed house, and whose early life diet contains high levels of allergenic foods has a greatly increased risk of developing allergies.

Why is allergy becoming more common?

The single most important risk factor for developing allergic disease is being born to a mother or father who has allergic disease him- or herself. However, there has been a marked rise in the number of people suffering from allergies within just one generation and, as we know that changes in the genetic make-up of our population cannot occur that quickly, other factors must be involved. These include the following.

Infant feeding

If babies are exposed to food allergens such as cows' milk and eggs early in life they are more likely to develop allergic disease. Breast-feeding does not entirely protect the infant because allergens from food eaten by the mother can be secreted in breast milk.

Although current Department of Health guidelines suggest that solid food should not be introduced before the age of six months, many babies are started on solids rather earlier. Our western diet contains increasing amounts of commercially prepared food containing preservatives and other chemicals, and decreasing quantities of certain foodstuffs such as fresh fruit and vegetables that contain protective antioxidants.

Antioxidants are substances that slow down the breakdown of another substance by oxidation. They can also mop up free radicals, molecules that could otherwise damage healthy DNA (genetic material). The most important antioxidants are vitamins A, C and E and selenium, with high levels being found in fresh fruit and vegetables.

Delaying the introduction of solid food appears to protect against allergies, especially eczema. The incidence of eczema by age two is directly related to the number of different solid foods taken by the baby before the age of four months. If a breast-feeding mother herself avoids highly allergenic food such as milk, eggs, peanuts and fish, an extra protective effect is seen, as all of these substances can pass into breast milk.

Other allergens

Exposure to high levels of air-borne allergens in very early life appears to increase an infant's risk of developing allergic disease. Babies born in spring when

Who develops allergies?

Allergies have a tendency to run in families. This is called atopy. Environmental factors also play a part in the development of allergic disorders. This is why not all members of a family are affected to the same extent.

Environment

Genetic factors

- Timing of first exposure to allergen

- Viral infection

- Tobacco smoke

- Allergenic foods

- Airborne allergens

- Household factors, e.g. dust mite

the pollen count is high are more likely to be allergic to plant pollens at age ten than children born at other times of the year. Similarly, babies exposed to pet allergens in very early life have an increased risk of allergy. Although sensitisation may occur at any age, the first year of life appears to be particularly relevant, and there is increasing evidence to show that exposures in mid and late pregnancy are also important.

Tobacco smoke

Exposure to tobacco smoke both before (via the mother's bloodstream) and after birth is strongly associated with the development of allergies and allergic disease, particularly asthma. Babies born to smoking mothers have raised levels of IgE in their blood at birth. Exposure to smoke after birth increases the risk – children living with a mother who smokes are four times as likely to develop wheezing and twice as likely to be admitted to hospital with chest illness as children living in non-smoking households. These children also have significantly reduced lung function by age seven. Passive tobacco smoke exposure is the strongest identified risk factor for the development of allergic disease and so it is particularly alarming to see that smoking is still most popular in young women of childbearing age.

Indoor environment

European children spend at least 90 per cent of their time indoors so the indoor environment is probably more important than all other geographical and outdoor environmental factors. Modern buildings tend to be well insulated and have poor levels of ventilation, and these factors appear to be a risk factor for the development of allergies. This may be the result of increased levels of chemical fumes from materials such as plastics and synthetic paints, high humidity leading to indoor mould growth and increased levels of house-dust mite allergen. These living conditions seem to exert a particularly powerful effect in atopic children, who are already at risk because of a family history of asthma.

Infections and antibiotics

Clear evidence is emerging that frequent viral and bacterial infections in early life may protect against the development of atopy and allergic diseases. Early life infections encourage the production of a chemical called interferon-gamma, which is found in higher levels in non-allergic people than in allergic people. If our children produce lower levels of interferon-gamma because we protect them from catching minor infections when they are young, we may be inadvertently increasing their chances of developing allergic disease. The overuse of antibiotics may have a similar effect.

In contrast, children who have a large number of older brothers and sisters, and who go to childcare centres where they mix with large numbers of other children (and their germs), are less likely to develop hay fever and asthma.

Immunisations

It is vital that we continue to protect our children from dangerous infections such as polio, tetanus, whooping cough, measles, mumps and rubella by the use of immunisations. Any theoretical benefit on the incidence of allergy that might result from not immunising is vastly outweighed by the harm done in leaving children vulnerable to catching these childhood infections; all of them are unpleasant and some can kill.

Finally

Our western diet, with the use of formula rather than breast milk and the early introduction of solid foods, in combination with our western lifestyle (early life exposure to tobacco smoke, high levels of plant and animal allergens, house-dust mite; living in poorly ventilated humid houses; having smaller families and delayed use of childcare centres), all conspire to increase the number of children in our population developing allergic problems.

KEY POINTS

■ An allergic reaction is an inappropriate and harmful response of your body's defence mechanisms to substances that are normally harmless

■ Sensitisation does not always occur the first time that your body meets a particular allergen, and a substance may be tolerated for many years before an allergy develops

■ Once you have become sensitised, even a tiny amount of allergen can produce an allergic response

■ Although atopy (genetic tendency towards allergy) is inherited, environmental factors, especially tobacco smoke exposure, also play a part in the development of allergic disorders

Which medical conditions are related to allergy?

A number of common and well-known conditions such as asthma, hay fever and eczema are allergic in nature. There are other less common but still important conditions, for example, urticaria and anaphylaxis, which are also caused by allergens.

Asthma

Asthma is the most common chronic disease of childhood, affecting about one in seven children. About one in ten adults has asthma. Asthma can develop at any age, even in elderly people, in whom it is often confused with bronchitis, which is an infection of the airways. To understand what happens in asthma, it helps to learn about the structure of the airways.

The normal airway has a delicate lining (epithelium) consisting of a number of different types of cells. These include cells that produce a lubricant (mucus) and cells with fine hair-like processes (cilia). These cilia move rhythmically to pass the mucus from the small airways upwards towards the back of the throat, where it is swallowed. It carries with it any dust particles and micro-organisms that have been breathed in.

Beneath the epithelium is a layer called the submucosa. Beneath the submucosa is a sheet of muscle that wraps around the airway which, when it contracts, makes the airways narrower.

Asthma is a chronic inflammation of the lining of the lung airways that leads to:

- swollen airway walls and narrowed air passages
- increased mucus production in the airways
- twitchy and oversensitive (hyperreactive) airway muscles.

The common symptoms of asthma are chest tightness, shortness of breath, wheeze and cough.

Narrowed swollen airways make it more difficult for air to move in and out of the lungs. This leads to wheezing. The lining of the airways is irritable, leading to episodes of coughing. As the airway wall muscles are hyperreactive, further airway narrowing can occur quite rapidly, producing sudden (acute) symptoms. There are often signs of other allergic diseases too.

Sometimes there is a clear link between symptoms and a trigger such as contact with an allergen, for example, when a person who is allergic to cats visits a cat-owning family and has an exacerbation of his or her wheezing and coughing. At other times, symptoms seem to occur for no particular reason. Common triggers to symptoms include:

- allergens, for example, pet dander, house-dust mite, mould spores

What happens during an asthma attack?

During an asthma attack, the muscle walls of the airway contract, causing the internal diameter to narrow. Increased mucus secretions and inflammation of the airways' inner linings cause further narrowing.

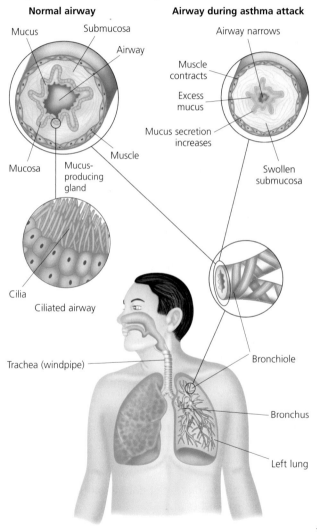

Normal airway

Mucus

Submucosa

Airway

Mucosa

Mucus-producing gland

Muscle

Cilia

Ciliated airway

Airway during asthma attack

Airway narrows

Muscle contracts

Excess mucus

Mucus secretion increases

Swollen submucosa

Trachea (windpipe)

Bronchiole

Bronchus

Left lung

- upper respiratory tract infections, for example, the common cold, particularly in children
- tobacco smoke
- high levels of air pollution
- sudden changes in air temperature
- exercise.

When more than one trigger is present, for example when going for a run alongside a busy road on a very cold day, their combined effect can be particularly potent.

Some young children with asthma appear well and symptom free most of the time, and develop asthma symptoms only when they meet one of their triggers. They then have an asthma attack, which may last a few hours or go on for days. Sometimes, long-term exposure to a trigger such as allergens or cigarette smoke leads to persistent symptoms as well. Removing the trigger often leads to a marked improvement.

The pattern tends to be different in older children and adults, who have persistent (chronic) symptoms as well as sudden worsening of their asthma in the form of asthma attacks.

Hay fever

Hay fever is a misleading term because hay has very little to do with causing the problem, and sufferers rarely have a fever. The medical term for hay fever is 'seasonal allergic rhinitis' – seasonal because it occurs only in certain months of the year and rhinitis meaning inflammation of the nose.

If you have seasonal hay fever, you are allergic to an allergen that is light enough to be carried in the air (an aeroallergen) and that is found only at particular times of year. A wide range of allergens can cause hay fever, including grass pollen, flower pollens, a wide variety of tree pollens and mould spores. You can be allergic to more than one allergen, so your symptoms might fluctuate throughout the pollen season.

If your hay fever symptoms go on all year, then your condition is called perennial allergic rhinitis, and the likely culprit is the house-dust mite, feathers or a pet allergen, for example, cat or dog dander. Although it is not a life-threatening condition, hay fever causes a great deal of misery. It is also very common, affecting up to a quarter of the population at some time during the year.

There might also be sleep disturbance leading to fatigue, lethargy and irritability. In addition, asthma, which often coexists with hay fever, can be worse.

These symptoms come from a localised allergic reaction in the nose, throat and eyes. Once an allergy to a particular aeroallergen has occurred, further contact with the allergen stimulates the cells lining your nose, throat and eyes to release histamine and other chemicals, causing the small blood vessels to enlarge and become leaky. Your eyes become itchy and watery, your nose becomes stuffed up and runny, and sneezing is a common problem. Some people find that they also have itchiness of the ears, caused by stimulation of a nerve linking the back of the throat and the ears.

As your nose is often blocked, your senses of smell and taste are affected. Swelling of the lining of your sinuses, the air-filled spaces in the bones of your face, can affect their drainage and cause sinusitis. On top of all these symptoms, sufferers often feel miserable,

What are the symptoms?

The symptoms of hay fever are:
- runny nose
- sneezing
- nasal congestion
- watery, red, itchy eyes
- itchy throat and nose
- impaired sense of smell
- headaches
- sore throat and hoarseness
- snoring
- dark circles under the eyes

irritable and listless, and many people find that their ability to work, drive and enjoy their social life is seriously impaired. Children with hay fever often find it difficult to perform well in end-of-year examinations that generally fall during the hay fever season.

Hay fever is rare in very young children. The most common time for it to start is between the ages of 6 and 25, and it is much less common in elderly people. Individuals who have previously suffered eczema or asthma are more at risk of developing hay fever.

The skin: eczema, dermatitis, urticaria and angio-oedema

The skin is the largest organ of the body and every day it is in direct contact with a vast array of different substances, including many allergens. It is not therefore surprising that the skin is frequently affected by allergic disease.

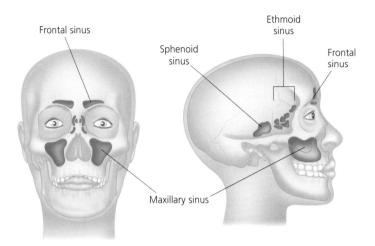

The sinuses are several air-filled cavities located in the skull bones around the eyes, cheeks and nose. Swelling of the lining of the sinuses can cause unpleasant symptoms.

What are the symptoms?

Common symptoms of skin allergies are:
- itchiness
- redness
- blisters
- weals
- skin thickening
- puffiness
- dry patches
- open weeping areas as a result of scratching

There are four main skin problems caused by allergy: eczema, contact dermatitis, urticaria and angio-oedema.

Eczema

The correct name for eczema is atopic dermatitis. This is a chronic (long-lasting and recurring) inflammatory skin condition that occurs in atopic individuals (see page 21). Up to 15 per cent of children develop eczema in childhood, and over 50 per cent of these children go on to develop asthma and 75 per cent of them develop hay fever. This is because eczema usually occurs in children who have inherited a tendency for allergic reaction from their parents (atopy).

A number of everyday factors can increase the likelihood of eczema developing. Exposure early in life to certain allergens such as eggs, cows' milk, pet dander and house-dust mite may increase the risk. At least 80 per cent of eczema sufferers have positive allergy tests to one or more allergens.

Eczema usually starts before the age of five years and, although it tends to improve over time, about 25 per cent of affected children continue to have eczema into adulthood.

Eczema causes itchy, red, raised lesions on the skin that can look blistered. They are often open and weeping as a result of scratching. Eventually the skin becomes thickened and scaly. The site of the lesions varies with age. In infants, eczema can cover the whole skin surface, although the nappy area is often spared. In older children and adults, eczema usually affects the neck, ankles, and inner aspects of the knees and elbows. Persistent scratching can cause patchy changes in the pigmentation of the skin, which can look darker

Typical example of atopic eczema

Eczema causes itchy, red, raised lesions of the skin that can look blistered. They are often open and weeping as a result of scratching.

or lighter. Also, chronic longstanding infection of the affected areas often occurs. The skin lesions follow a relapsing course, with bad episodes often being followed by periods when symptoms subside.

Once eczema has developed, certain triggers can make it worse. These include:

- diet – such as eating a trigger food
- chemicals – for example, in washing powders (particularly biological ones that include enzymes), skin creams, cosmetics, soaps and shampoos
- stress and anxiety

The location of eczema varies with age

Infants – whole body except bottom and groin

Children – neck, ankles, legs and arms

The location of eczema varies with age
(contd)

Adults – neck, ankles, inner aspects of the knees and elbows

- the weather – particularly cold weather
- airborne allergens such as pollen, pet allergens and house-dust mite.

Changing to feather bedding, acquiring a new furry pet and high pollen levels can all make eczema worse. Remember that manufacturers sometimes change the formulation of their products, so a product that you have used without a problem in the past may suddenly cause your skin to get worse. You may not be reacting to something that you have put on your own skin – enough of a product to cause an allergic reaction can be transferred by hugging and kissing.

Allergic contact dermatitis

Contact dermatitis occurs when the skin is in contact with a chemical that can act as an irritant or an allergen. Most contact dermatitis is not allergic, and is caused by substances that are not allergens but irritants – even the least allergic one of us can develop non-allergic dermatitis if sufficient irritant is applied to our skin for long enough.

Only about 20 per cent of all cases of contact dermatitis are caused by allergens and this problem is known as allergic contact dermatitis. This happens once an individual has been sensitised to that particular substance. Allergic contact dermatitis is more common in atopic (inherited predisposition to allergy) individuals (see page 21), and is found most often in adults, being rare in children and elderly people.

Sensitisation usually takes several days to develop. If the chemical is then in contact with the skin again, a reaction will develop within 48 hours. This time delay can make the identification of the cause very difficult.

Allergic contact dermatitis is the most common work-related illness. People in certain jobs are more at risk, particularly hairdressers, cleaners and factory workers. It is more common in people with fair skin, and in women, probably because they have more contact with the chemicals found in household cleaners and use more skin preparations than men.

The skin lesions in allergic contact dermatitis can look very similar to those in eczema. Blistering of the surface of the skin can be followed by thickening and scaling. There is often intense itching. However, only the parts of the body exposed to the allergen are affected. Over half of all cases involve the hands. The outline of the

Contact dermatitis

Nickel-plated jewellery

Nickel allergy is probably the most common cause of allergic contact dermatitis.

area involved might suggest the cause – the round imprint of a watch on the wrist, a rectangle on the skin the same size as a sticking plaster, or a rash on the part of a face on which a particular cosmetic is used. This is in contrast to the lesions seen in eczema, which are not well demarcated.

Substances most commonly causing contact dermatitis are nickel, soaps and detergents, food substances, preservatives, fragrances, lanolin, formaldehyde and potassium dichromate. Plants such as chrysanthemums and plant-derived materials such as latex may also be to blame.

Nickel allergy is probably the most common cause of allergic contact dermatitis, with at least ten per cent of the population being affected. Nickel is found in jewellery, zips and buttons on jeans.

Urticaria and angio-oedema

When an immediate allergic reaction happens in the skin, it becomes itchy and raised weals occur which look like nettle rash. Redness and swelling around the weals can also be seen. These changes are caused by acute (rapid-onset) allergic inflammation, which is called urticaria. Acute urticaria affects as many as 20 per cent of the population at some time in their lives. It is usually short-lived and gets better without any treatment, although in rare cases the urticaria can persist for weeks.

When the same type of reaction occurs in deeper layers of the skin, the reaction is called angio-oedema. In this there is little or no itching but the swelling might be quite painful. Although urticaria can happen virtually anywhere on the skin, angio-oedema usually involves the face and tongue, where it may cause serious problems with breathing.

Example of urticaria

Urticaria.

A wide range of different factors can cause urticaria and angio-oedema. These include:

- direct contact with allergen (including foods, colourings, preservatives, chemicals and drugs), by skin contact, inhalation, injection or ingestion
- infections
- physical stimuli – such as cold, pressures, vibration and sunlight
- exercise (rarely).

Example of angio-oedema

Angio-oedema.

Food allergies

Although unpleasant reactions to foods are common, not all of these are caused by allergy. As many as 20 per cent of the population believe that they are allergic to one or more foodstuffs, but, on formal diagnostic testing, fewer than one in ten of these people has true food allergy, putting the true figure at about two per cent. The rest are not imagining their symptoms, which are real – they may be caused by the food in question but it is not acting as an allergen.

Allergy, aversion, intolerance and sensitivity

In a large study enquiring about food allergy in 7,500 households, 20 per cent of households reported that at least one family member had food allergy. However, when these individuals were scientifically tested (using a double-blind, placebo-controlled challenge, see page

73) only between 1.4 and 1.8 per cent of adults had true food allergy. The symptoms in all the others may have been caused by food aversion, food intolerance or food sensitivity.

Food aversion
People with food aversion have had a previous unpleasant experience with a particular food and believe that whenever they eat the same food again they will have the same unpleasant reaction. This is not so, but, because they believe that it will happen, they feel unwell even when they see or think of the food in question.

Food intolerance
In food intolerance, unpleasant symptoms occur after eating a food because the body cannot handle that food adequately. For example, some people have unpleasant symptoms of bloating, crampy abdominal pain and diarrhoea when they drink milk or eat products made from milk. This is because they do not produce sufficient quantities of the bowel enzyme that digests the milk sugar, lactose. Small quantities of milk can often be tolerated, but larger quantities lead to these symptoms. This is not because of an allergy, in which even tiny amounts can lead to quite severe symptoms, but is the result of intolerance of lactose. Symptoms can be avoided by eliminating milk and milk products from the diet.

Food sensitivity
Food sensitivity occurs when you are more than usually sensitive to certain properties of a food. The type of reaction can be predicted from the food's chemical composition. For example, some people are very

sensitive to the caffeine found in coffee and tea – they feel anxious and have marked tremor of their hands after taking even small quantities.

It is important to distinguish intolerance, sensitivity, aversion and allergy, so that you receive the most effective form of treatment for your condition and understand how it may affect you in the future. For example, whereas small children often outgrow their milk allergy, if you suffer from lactose intolerance your condition will probably stay with you all your life.

What foods cause allergic reactions?

In young children, the most common food allergies are to cows' milk and eggs. In later childhood, fish, shellfish, peanuts and tree nuts are the most common allergens. Some allergies, particularly cows' milk allergy, may improve with time; others such as peanut allergy generally stay with you. Cows' milk allergy occurs in between two and five per cent of infants with up to 80 per cent of these infants losing their allergy by the age of five.

Children allergic to cows' milk are almost always allergic to sheep and goats' milk, and so these should not be used as a substitute. Soy-based milks should be used instead, and are well tolerated by most infants.

What are the symptoms?

Food allergy can cause a range of allergic symptoms in a number of different parts of the body. These symptoms may be mild, moderate or may be severe and occur within minutes of the exposure.

Mild

- Itchy skin rash – similar to nettle rash (urticaria).

Moderate

- Swelling of the lips, tongue and face (angio-oedema)
- Swelling of the throat and larynx (voice box).

Severe

- Wheezing and shortness of breath
- Breathing difficulties
- Severe life-threatening collapse with shock (anaphylaxis).

Other symptoms can come on after a delay of a few hours, including:

- nausea
- abdominal pains
- vomiting and diarrhoea
- worsening of eczema.

Peanut allergy

The number of people affected by allergy to peanuts is rising. Peanut allergy was rare 10 years ago, but has trebled over the last four years and now affects one in 70 children. This problem has received a great deal of attention in the media in recent years, resulting at least in part from the small but increasing number of deaths occurring in young people caused by peanut allergy.

If you have asthma, especially if your asthma is poorly controlled, you are more at risk of having a severe allergic reaction to food.

The peanut (*Arachis hypogea*) is not a true nut but a legume (a seed that grows in a pod), related to the lentil and pea families. Another name for it is ground nut. Peanuts are a cheap source of protein and are

Food allergy

- Unpleasant reactions to foods are common and allergy is only one of many causes
- Symptoms of food allergy can range from mild itchy rashes to life-threatening anaphylaxis
- The most common foods causing allergy in the UK are cows' milk, hens' eggs, peanuts, fish and shellfish
- The best way of managing food allergy is to avoid the allergen

used widely in the world both as food and as one of the largest sources of edible oil.

Peanut oil is used in cooking, as well as in a wide range of cosmetic preparations such as soaps and shampoos, and in medical skin care products. In the past, peanut oil was used in many infant milk formulas, but, in response to the rapid rise in allergy to peanut, this practice has now been stopped.

The allergens responsible for peanut allergy are stable to heat and not destroyed by cooking. Although good quality distilled peanut (ground nut) oil does not contain any protein and is therefore not a risk for peanut-allergic patients, cold pressed oils can contain significant amounts of protein and can cause an allergic reaction. As peanuts are used in a wide range of items to which babies are exposed, sensitisation can occur early in life. The resulting allergy is usually life long.

Allergic reactions to peanuts can be classed as mild, moderate or severe. If itchy skin rashes (hives, urticaria) are the only symptom, it is a mild reaction. A moderate reaction might involve swelling of the face, tightening

Ingredients

Whole Wheat, Malt Extract. Sugar, Salt, Colour: Annatto, Preservative: Sulphur, Dioxide, Niacin, Iron, Riboflavin (B2), Thiamine (B1), Folic Acid

Nutritional Information

	per 100g	per 37.5g serving
Energy	140kj	540kj
	340cal	128cal
Protein	11.2g	4.2g
Carbohydrate	67.6g	25.4g
(of which sugars)	(4.7g)	(1.8g)
Fat	2.7g	1.0g
(of which saturates)	(0.6g)	(0.2g)
Fibre	10.5g	3.9g
Soluble	3.2g	1.2g
Insoluble	7.3g	0.2g
Sodium	0.4g	0.2g

Vitamins	per 100g	per 37.5g serving
Thiamine (B1)	1.2mg85%RDA	0.4mg32%RDA
Riboflavin (B2)	1.4mg85%RDA	0.5mg32%RDA
Niacin	15.3mg85%RDA	5.7mg32%RDA
Folic Acid	170.0mg85%RDA	63.8mg32%RDA
Iron	11.9mg85%RDA	4.5mg32%RDA

An average serving of 37.5g of **cereal** will provide 32% of the recommended daily allowance (RDA) for the average adult of the vitamins and iron listed

Made in England by ANOTHER PLC.

BEST BEFORE END: DEC 2020

CEREAL

RICH IN CARBOHYDRATE

900g

NEW

900g

The nutritional panel on food packaging will help you avoid the substances causing your symptoms.

of the throat and breathing difficulties other than wheezing.

A severe reaction (called an anaphylactic reaction) would include wheezing, abdominal pain and circulatory collapse, with blueness of the lips and tongue. Peanut allergy is the most common cause of severe allergic reactions (anaphylaxis) in the USA and possibly now also in the UK.

In 90 per cent of peanut-allergic individuals, the allergic reaction can be caused by a very small amount of peanuts (less than one nut). In over 50 per cent of sufferers, the symptoms start immediately after exposure and in 76 per cent within five minutes. In general, children suffer milder reactions than adults. Most peanut-allergic individuals suffer either mild or moderate reactions, severe reactions occurring in only seven per cent. Severe reactions are more common in those who also have asthma.

The best way of diagnosing peanut allergy is from the answers given to questions about your medical past (the clinical history), in combination with skin-prick testing (see 'Diagnosing your allergies', page 66).

The size of the reaction on skin-prick testing to peanuts is related to the severity of the reaction. Skin-prick testing is more sensitive than measuring the levels of specific antibodies (specific IgE) in the blood, and these antibody levels do not tend to mirror the severity of the allergic reaction.

Once peanut allergy has been diagnosed, it is vital that all forms of peanuts are excluded from your diet. However, this is easier said than done! At least 50 per cent of people known to have peanut allergy have at least one accidental exposure each year. As a result of this, if you have peanut allergy you must AT ALL TIMES carry with you the right treatment to combat an allergic reaction (see 'Use of the EpiPen', page 63).

Sesame allergy

Sesame seeds are an extremely potent source of allergen. Sesame is used extensively in the food industry, both in its unprocessed form as a decoration for bread and other baked products and in a wide range of processed foods, pharmaceutical products, toiletries and cosmetics.

If you have sesame allergy, eating out may be a major problem – both the seeds and the oil produced from them must be avoided, because sesame oil is unrefined and may contain considerable amounts of sesame protein.

Sesame allergy was first reported in 1950 but initially very few cases were diagnosed. There has been a considerable rise in the numbers of people developing sesame allergy in the last decade. In one recent study of Australian children, sesame allergy was more common than allergy to tree nuts, although significantly less common than peanut allergy. In the UK, sesame allergy is believed to affect approximately one in every 2,000 people.

If you are allergic to sesame seeds, the mainstay of management is the avoidance of foods and other preparations containing sesame.

Allergies at work

Since the link was made between certain health problems and particular jobs, a number of Government Acts have tried to ensure that employees' working conditions are safe. A large number of health problems, some of which are allergic in origin, are still caused by contact with certain substances in the workplace. Allergies to such substances (occupational allergies) occur in both atopic (inherited predisposition to allergy) and non-atopic individuals, being only slightly more common in those with asthma, eczema or hay fever. Many of the problem substances encountered at work do not cause allergy but act as irritants instead. These should be avoided by ensuring good workplace ventilation, by wearing or providing barrier clothing, or by substituting non-irritant alternatives.

However, there are over 200 substances that can cause allergic sensitisation leading to occupational asthma, and at least as many causing skin allergies. About 900,000 working days a year are lost in the UK because of occupational dermatitis. Occupational asthma accounts for two per cent of all adult asthma, with over 1,000 new cases per year.

Workplace allergies are becoming more common. Until 1979 only two cases of latex allergy had been described. Now, eight per cent of health-care workers are allergic to latex. Many of these have had to change their job. Most large hospitals now have a latex-free operating theatre for use by latex-allergic patients who might have a dangerous allergic reaction to the numerous pieces of medical equipment containing latex found in ordinary operating theatre suites.

Employers have a legal duty to protect their employees from hazards in the workplace and these include contact with allergic sensitisers. If you develop any work-related symptoms, act straight away. Provided that an occupational allergy is diagnosed early and, from then on, the problem substances are avoided, there is a reasonable chance that the symptoms will disappear. However, if an allergy is allowed to become long standing, avoidance of the cause may only improve the symptoms and they may not disappear completely.

If you suspect that you have developed an occupational allergy, it is important for you to contact your work's doctor, your employment medical adviser or your general practitioner, so that you may be referred for further tests and specialist advice.

The most common substances causing allergy encountered in the workplace are latex, formaldehyde, soaps and detergents, food substances, potassium dichromate (found in many substances used in the building industry and in tanning leather), dyes and the chemicals used in hairdressing.

How to avoid allergic reactions in the workplace

- Avoid contact with materials that carry a manufacturer's hazard warning
- Avoid damage to your skin from rough or abrasive work with your hands
- Always wash your hands properly after handling any potential irritant, but avoid getting your hands excessively wet, because damp skin is a less effective barrier
- Protect your hands from solvents, glue, grease, oil and corrosive chemicals by using barrier creams, after-wash creams and gloves
- Do not use solvents to remove substances from your hands as they themselves can cause dermatitis
- Use all protective apparatus supplied by your employer
- Avoid breathing in dust and fumes
- Report any problems to your line manager
- Encourage your colleagues to report their own work-related problems to their line manager

Drug allergies

There are a number of different ways in which drugs can cause adverse reactions, and not all of these are allergy related. It is important to diagnose accurately whether or not allergy is responsible for your symptoms because the medical management and long-term outlook of allergic and non-allergic reactions differ considerably.

Not all drugs can cause allergy. Those that do most frequently are penicillin, other antibiotics, barbiturates, local anaesthetics and treatments that involve the injection of large molecules (such as insulin, some vaccines and some antisera made to treat the victims of bites by venomous creatures).

Drug allergy is becoming more common, and now accounts for five per cent of all hospital admission. A drug allergy can take many forms, including urticaria, contact dermatitis (from topically applied drugs), anaphylaxis, and severe generalised inflammation of the skin and the lining of the mouth and eyes (Stevens–Johnson syndrome).

A number of factors increase your risk of developing a drug allergy. These include:

- a current infection
- a family history of drug allergy
- a personal history of previous drug allergy
- diseases affecting your immune system, especially HIV
- if a number of different drugs are given in combination
- multiple courses or continuous use of a drug.

Although being atopic does not increase your likelihood of developing a drug allergy, it does increase your risk of having a severe reaction.

KEY POINTS

- Asthma is the most common chronic disease of childhood, affecting about one in seven children

- A wide range of allergens may be responsible for causing hay fever

- At least 80 per cent of eczema sufferers have positive allergy tests to one or more allergens

- Contact dermatitis occurs when the skin is exposed to an irritant or an allergen

- Urticaria and angio-oedema are two forms of immediate allergic reactions affecting the skin

- As many as twenty per cent of the population believe that they are allergic to one or more foodstuffs, but only one in ten of these have true food allergy

- Once peanut allergy has been diagnosed, it is vital that all forms of peanuts are excluded from the diet

- Employers have a legal duty to protect their employees from hazards in the workplace and these include contact with allergic sensitisers

Anaphylaxis

What is anaphylaxis?

Anaphylaxis is the most severe type of allergic reaction. Anaphylactic reactions are potentially fatal because they occur within minutes of the allergen exposure, affect many different systems of the body, and without treatment progress with frightening rapidity.

Each year, one in every 3,500 people in the UK will have an anaphylactic reaction, and about 30 people will die each year, mainly young adults. Admissions to hospital for anaphylaxis have increased sevenfold over the last ten years.

In anaphylaxis, the allergic reaction is widespread within the body, including the skin, the respiratory tract (mouth, nose, windpipe and lungs), the gastrointestinal tract (mouth, throat, stomach and intestine) and the cardiovascular system (heart and blood vessels). People who have asthma or other allergies are at particular risk from anaphylactic reactions, especially if their asthma is poorly controlled.

Symptoms of anaphylaxis

Anaphylactic reactions result from an exposure to an allergen to which a person is already sensitised. Instead of a localised reaction such as those described in the previous chapter, this exposure produces a whole-body reaction. The widespread triggering of basophils and mast cells by IgE (see page 11) results in large-scale release of inflammatory mediators such as histamine and leukotrienes, which cause increased leakiness of the small blood vessels throughout the whole body. Fluid rapidly leaks from these small blood vessels into the tissues. This causes swelling within many body parts, which can interfere with normal body functioning, and loss of blood volume, causing blood pressure to fall.

These changes result in the following symptoms:

- generalised itchiness, including itchiness of the skin, nose, eyes and throat
- flushing (reddening) of the skin
- urticaria and angio-oedema (see pages 42–3)
- hoarseness and difficulty in swallowing, because of swelling in the throat
- chest tightness and wheeze, caused by swelling and narrowing of the airways
- a fall in blood pressure causing a rapid weak pulse and a feeling of faintness
- difficulty in breathing and blueness of the lips
- nausea, vomiting and abdominal pain
- in severe cases, respiratory and circulatory collapse and death.

Triggers of anaphylaxis
The most common triggers to anaphylactic reactions are:

- bee and wasp stings
- foods, especially shellfish, peanuts, nuts, eggs and fish

- drugs, particularly antibiotics
- vaccines, especially tetanus anti-toxin.

In a few cases, no cause of the anaphylactic reaction is discovered.

Diagnosis

Once an individual has recovered from a severe allergic reaction, it is important to identify the trigger that caused it, because one of the main management strategies is the avoidance of that trigger in the future.

In many cases a particular trigger will be fairly obvious, but in others the cause will be a mystery. Careful questioning by an allergy expert will often unravel the cause. Skin-prick testing is the diagnostic test of choice – in most cases a direct challenge test is too dangerous in case it triggers another severe allergic reaction (see 'Diagnosing your allergies', pages 66–82).

Management of anaphylaxis
Specialist clinics

Everyone who suffers anaphylaxis or a severe allergic reaction should be referred by the hospital in which they are treated or by their GP to an allergy specialist, a hospital consultant trained in the diagnosis and management of allergy. A list of allergy specialists is available from the British Society for Allergy and Clinical Immunology (see 'Useful information', page 133).

Trigger avoidance

If the trigger to anaphylaxis is known, it should be scrupulously avoided. If the trigger is a food, the help of a dietitian may be very useful in helping you to avoid that food in the future. Your GP or allergy specialist can refer you. Even very small traces of the problem food can trigger a reaction, and in severe cases skin contact with the allergen (for example, even being kissed by someone who has recently eaten food containing the allergen) or breathing in air containing tiny particles of it may be enough to cause a reaction. (See pages 44–51 for avoidance of food allergens.)

There are many practical things that you can do to reduce the risk of being stung (see 'Treatment of allergic disease', page 83).

What you should do if you are stung by a bee or wasp – mild-to-moderate reactions

- Keep calm, and if possible do not walk or run around because this will rapidly spread the allergen around the body and put you at more risk of a severe reaction.

- If the sting remains embedded in your skin, remove it with tweezers, making sure not to squeeze the poison sac, which is a dark pouch that is at the back of the sting.

- Cool the affected area, if possible with an ice pack or packet of frozen vegetables, covered with a towel or tea towel so as not to burn your skin.

- For pain, take a pain-killer such as paracetamol or ibuprofen (ibuprofen is an anti-inflammatory as well as a pain-killer so is preferable, but take whichever you have to hand). If you develop anything more than mild local swelling, take an antihistamine (available over the counter from your chemist).

- If the reaction doesn't subside and you develop more severe symptoms, follow your emergency treatment plan (see page 60).

Emergency treatment plan

You should prepare an emergency treatment plan so that you and those around you know exactly what to do if you experience a severe allergic reaction. Don't think this won't happen to you. Approximately half of all people at risk of anaphylaxis are accidentally exposed to the trigger allergen that could cause a life-threatening allergic reaction each year. If you act quickly, you will be able to reduce the severity of the reaction greatly.

Carry with you an **information card** with your name, a brief description of your allergy and what treatment you may need if you have a severe allergic reaction, your address and emergency contact numbers for close relatives. Make it clear that you have a SERIOUS medical problem and state that anyone helping you should call an ambulance by dialling 999 immediately. You may also wish to wear a piece of medical identification jewellery (see 'Treatment of allergic disease', page 83 and 'Useful information', page 133).

Example of medical identity jewellery.

You should carry a copy of this plan with your emergency drug. Further copies should be given to appropriate colleagues and carers such as work colleagues, teachers and close friends. Special plans should be devised for children with severe allergy, and sample plans are available from the Anaphylaxis Campaign and Allergy UK (see 'Useful information', page 133).

Treatment for severe allergic reactions
Antihistamine medications

These should be taken as soon as you realise that you are having an allergic reaction. Common preparations include chlorpheniramine (Piriton), cetirizine (Zirtek) and loratadine (Clarityn). These drugs block the effect of histamine, a substance released by the mast cells, which causes many of the symptoms of allergy – they may prevent a full-blown anaphylactic reaction from developing. Use chlorpheniramine if you have it, as it begins to work more quickly than the others.

Epinephrine (adrenaline)

If you are having a severe allergic reaction, epinephrine will temporarily reverse some of the life-threatening effects and allow you enough time to seek urgent medical attention.

In the UK, the name adrenaline has been superseded by epinephrine. Epinephrine works quickly when injected by counteracting the effects of the chemicals released during an anaphylactic reaction. It relaxes the airways, narrows the small blood vessels, effectively increases the blood volume, stimulates the heart and increases the blood pressure.

If you are at risk of an anaphylactic reaction you should carry epinephrine for injection with you at all times. You should always carry two injectors because the effects of the first injection may begin to wear off before you reach medical help, in which case you will need a second injection.

Remember that epinephrine only buys you time – it is not a treatment for the severe allergic reaction. You will still require expert medical help – dial 999 immediately and go to an accident and emergency department as soon as possible.

You should learn how to administer the injections, and should also teach relatives and close friends. In the case of a child, all the child's carers (including school-teachers) should know how and when to administer the epinephrine. Epinephrine and antihistamines can be used together without problems.

The most commonly used device for injectable epinephrine in the UK is the EpiPen. This is very easy to use, and you should carry two pens with you everywhere you go. The best way to do this is to 'wear' them on your body in some way – in a pocket or a bumbag – rather than putting them in a bag, from which you might be separated at times during the day.

If you think you may be developing a severe allergic reaction, use your epinephrine pen EARLY. Do not wait until you are sure – the dose of epinephrine will do you no harm, even if you turn out to be wrong and you do not develop a reaction. However, failing to use epinephrine when you should puts you at risk of having the worst kind of allergic reaction, which could kill you. If in doubt, use the epinephrine!

Safety cap protects the needle and firing device

Measured epinephrine dose

The most commonly used device for injectable epinephrine in the UK is the EpiPen.

Use of the EpiPen

How to administer the injection

- Remove the EpiPen from the carrying case
- Never put your fingers, thumbs or hands over the black tip
- Grasp the EpiPen, forming a fist around the unit, with the black tip facing down
- Pull off the grey safety cap with your other hand
- Place the black tip level with your upper outer thigh (it is not necessary to remove your clothes unless they are very thick and bulky)
- Swing the pen back then jab it firmly into the outer thigh until it clicks
- Hold the pen in place for 10 seconds
- Remove the pen and massage the injection site gently for 10 seconds
- Call 999 and seek medical advice *immediately*
- If allergic symptoms do not start to improve, give a second injection of epinephrine
- Remember: carry two EpiPens with you at all times

Tips and precautions

Keep your EpiPen auto-injector at room temperature until the marked expiry date, at which point the unit should be replaced. It should not be refrigerated; refrigeration for extended periods may cause the unit to malfunction. Nor should the EpiPen auto-injector be exposed to extreme heat, such as in the glove compartment or boot of a car during the summer.

Use of the EpiPen (contd)

Do not expose your auto-injector to direct sunlight; light and heat can cause epinephrine to degrade, turning brown. This shortens the usable life of the product.

The best way to protect your auto-injector is to keep it in the plastic tube in which it comes. Do not put anything else, for example the patient information leaflet, in the tube, as this may prevent you removing the EpiPen when you need it.

Check your EpiPen auto-injector periodically through the viewing window of the unit to make sure that the solution is clear and colourless. If the solution appears brown, or if a red flag shows in the window, replace the unit immediately.

Regardless of the colour of the epinephrine, always replace your auto-injector with a fresh unit before the expiry date.

Seek medical help

If you need to use epinephrine you should call an ambulance IMMEDIATELY. A mobile phone may be a useful extra to have with you. Even though your prompt recognition and treatment of the allergic reaction may prevent anaphylaxis developing, you must go to an accident and emergency department where you will be observed for at least four hours to make sure that the reaction does not progress.

Remember, the effects of epinephrine do not last long – after 10–30 minutes you may need another dose. As each EpiPen contains only one dose of epinephrine, once you have used a pen you must get a new one from your doctor immediately.

KEY POINTS

- Anaphylaxis is the most severe type of allergic reaction and can be life threatening

- The most common triggers to anaphylactic reactions are foods (especially shellfish, peanuts, nuts, eggs and fish), bee and wasp stings, and drugs (particularly antibiotics)

- Anyone who has suffered anaphylaxis or a severe allergic reaction should be referred to an allergy specialist

- If the trigger to anaphylaxis is known, it should be scrupulously avoided

- Prepare and carry an emergency treatment plan

- Carry your EpiPen with you at all times and make sure you and others know how to use it

Diagnosing your allergies

How to get a diagnosis

If you think that you might have an allergy, it is important that your condition is accurately diagnosed. If it is an allergy, the correct treatment can be prescribed and a management plan worked out. If the problem is not the result of an allergy, you are then free to find out what the real cause is. This chapter describes each of the different allergy tests, with details of when each test might be needed, and a discussion of their advantages and disadvantages.

Your doctor will start by asking you to give a detailed account of your allergic reactions, your past medical history, your home and school/work environment, and your relevant family medical history. After performing a physical examination, he will almost certainly want to do at least one test. If you have suffered an allergic reaction but do not know what the cause was, the test will attempt to discover the allergen responsible. Even if you know the cause of your allergic reaction, the diagnosis may need to be confirmed by some form of allergy test, particularly if the allergic reaction was severe.

The treatment for an allergic condition may involve long-lasting, time-consuming or expensive treatments and so it is as well to verify the cause beforehand. Allergy tests can also be helpful if there is any confusion about whether your problem is caused by a true allergy or whether it might be caused by an intolerance or sensitivity. Workplace allergies may have legal implications, and must always be verified by formal allergy testing.

The results of allergy tests must be interpreted by an expert, who will also consider the precise details of your problem. This is because allergy tests do not always provide a clear yes/no answer – rather they provide a clue in the clinical puzzle. As a result of this, I would not recommend that you have allergy tests performed by a commercial organisation because they are unable to interpret the results in the light of your clinical history and advise you appropriately.

Choosing the right test

There is no such thing as a perfect test, and each one has advantages and disadvantages.

Every test used for diagnosing your allergies should be:

- relevant (includes the likely culprits)
- standardised (so that the results done in one centre can be related to those done in another)
- repeatable (so that results done on different occasions will be similar)
- specific (the test is positive only in people with that allergy)
- sensitive (the test does not falsely show as negative a test that should be positive).

No single allergy test fulfils all these criteria, but by choosing the best tests for each individual, the majority of allergic problems can be accurately diagnosed.

Which test is right for you will depend on the details of your allergic reaction – for example, how old you are, which part of your body is affected, what the likely cause is, how severe the reaction is.

If your problem proves particularly difficult to sort out, you should ask your doctor to refer you to an NHS allergy specialist – this is the only way you can get to see one. A list of allergy specialists in the UK can be obtained from the British Society for Allergy and Clinical Immunology (see 'Useful information', page 133).

Skin-prick tests

Direct skin testing is the most commonly used diagnostic test for allergy. The skin test is a way of challenging your body with an allergen to see whether you respond. This is an easy and localised test and is a very sensitive way to demonstrate the presence of a true allergic reaction. Skin-prick testing is very safe and adverse events are extremely rare. However, individuals at high risk of experiencing a severe allergic reaction should be skin tested in a hospital setting. You must tell the person doing the skin tests if you are on any medications because treatment with antihistamines, corticosteroids and certain antidepressants may interfere with the tests. Skin testing can also be unreliable in very young and elderly people.

Skin tests are usually done on the inside aspect of your forearm, but the skin of the back is often used in small children. The sites for testing are labelled with a pen and a single drop of a concentrated extract of

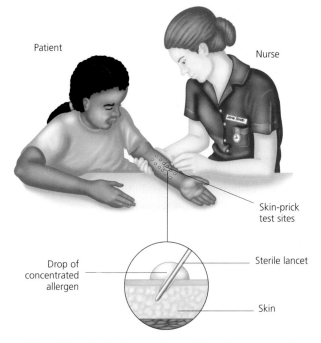

Patient

Nurse

Skin-prick
test sites

Drop of
concentrated
allergen

Sterile lancet

Skin

Skin-prick testing involves placing a drop of concentrated
allergen on the skin. The skin is then punctured through the
drop. A positive reaction to the allergen is shown by a pale
raised bump.

one of the chosen allergens is placed at each site.
The surface layer of your skin is gently punctured
through the drop using a sterile lancet (an instrument
with a small sharp prong one millimetre long). The whole
process is repeated using a new lancet for each allergen
being tested. Any allergen left on your skin is then
blotted with an absorbent tissue and after 10 minutes
the diameters of the resulting reactions are measured.
A positive result is shown by a weal (a pale raised
bump), which may be itchy and may be surrounded by
an area of redness.

As well as testing with allergens, two further pricks are done using a saline solution (negative control) and a histamine solution (a positive control) in order to test the reliability of the procedure.

The response to the saline solution should be negative in everyone. If you have a positive result this shows that your skin is very sensitive and that testing will not be reliable.

The response to histamine should be positive in everyone. If you have a negative result, your skin is being prevented from reacting normally, perhaps because of a drug you are taking and, again, testing will not be reliable.

Skin-prick testing is painless, and even young children tolerate the procedure very well. Positive reactions may be itchy but the itch generally lasts less than an hour.

Skin-prick testing is a very sensitive test, so if you have a negative reaction you can be fairly certain you do not have that allergy. However, a positive reaction does not always mean that you have a current allergy. It may be that you have a hidden or latent allergy that is not causing you problems now but that might have done so in the past or may do so in the future.

Skin-prick testing is a simple, quick and inexpensive form of testing and many different allergens can be tested at the same time, although there might not be enough space on your arm for more than 16.

Patch testing

This test is used in cases of contact dermatitis where allergy is suspected. It is generally performed on the skin of your back, and it is important that an area of clear skin, free of any disease, is used. It is a relatively

Metal disc containing the allergen

Patient

Positive test reaction

Surgical tape

After 48 hours the discs are removed

A patch test puts test allergens into small metal discs that are taped on to the skin of the back. The discs are left for 48 hours and then removed, and the underlying skin examined for reaction.

simple and safe form of testing but, in severe cases, itching or blistering may develop as a response to the tests.

Test allergens in appropriate concentrations are mixed with white soft paraffin (which allows them to penetrate the skin surface more easily) and then spread on to metal discs the size of a one pence piece. These discs are placed on your skin, covered with an adhesive dressing and left in place for 48 hours. The discs are then removed and discarded and your skin is examined for any redness, swelling or blistering. Your skin is then re-examined after a further 48 hours.

The interpretation of the results of this form of testing is not easy, and requires a thorough knowledge of the materials being used and of your personal allergy history. When carefully done, patch testing can provide very helpful information for the diagnosis of contact dermatitis.

Specific IgE measurements (RAST)

If a person is allergic to something, they should have specific IgE antibodies to that allergen in their blood. These allergy antibodies can be measured in the blood using a **r**adio**a**llergo**s**orbent **t**est (RAST). This test can confirm that your immune system has produced increased levels of IgE against a suspected allergen, for example, house-dust mite.

For this test, a small blood sample must be taken from a vein, usually from your arm, using a fine needle and small syringe. The sample is analysed by a

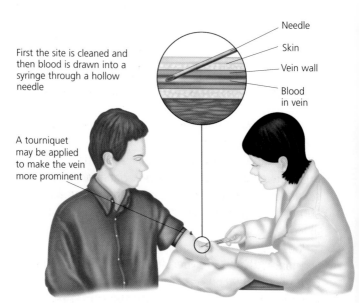

First the site is cleaned and then blood is drawn into a syringe through a hollow needle

Needle

Skin

Vein wall

Blood in vein

A tourniquet may be applied to make the vein more prominent

Specific allergy antibodies can be measured in the blood using a RAST to confirm that your immune system has produced increased levels of IgE against a suspect allergen.

specialist laboratory, which can generally provide results within a few days.

This test is particularly useful when skin-prick testing is impossible, perhaps because the patient is unable to stop their antihistamine medications without their allergic disease getting very much worse. Extensive eczema or dermatitis also makes skin-prick testing impractical. Again, careful interpretation of the results of RAST is important because positive tests can occur in people without an allergy, and negative tests can occasionally occur in people who do have that specific allergy.

Challenge tests

Occasionally the best way of diagnosing and confirming an allergy is to provoke an allergic reaction by deliberately exposing the person to the suspected allergen, but by doing this in a careful and controlled way. Anyone performing these tests should be well equipped to deal with any allergic reaction that might occur.

The allergen should be given in an appropriate way, for example, if wheezing or asthma is the problem, the allergen should be inhaled. If food allergy is suspected, the allergen should be swallowed. These forms of testing should never be used in a patient who has suffered a severe allergic reaction or anaphylaxis to the allergen.

Ideally both allergen and dummy (placebo) substances should be used and neither the individual being tested nor the tester should know which is which – this is called a 'double-blind placebo-controlled' challenge. A third person prepares the substances and keeps the records. The test is done in this way so that no one involved in the tests can be influenced by any prior beliefs that the person might have.

This form of test can be used when food allergy is suspected but the cause is not clear. For example, when several different foods have given a positive result on skin-prick testing, it might be unclear which of these foods is causing your symptoms. The results of a double-blind food challenge are usually very clear and, if a food does not give rise to symptoms, allergy can generally be ruled out. This type of test should NEVER be attempted at home, because it may result in a severe allergic reaction.

Lung function testing

Various forms of lung function tests can be used in making the diagnosis of asthma and in monitoring a patient's progress, particularly after changes in treatment.

The most common form of testing is the measurement of peak expiratory flow. Peak expiratory flowmeters (peak flowmeters) are small hand-held devices that measure the flow of air from your lungs. The harder you are able to blow, the higher the reading.

If you have asthma, your peak flow levels are likely to be lower than those of someone with normal lungs, but, in addition, the readings will vary more both during each day and from one day to another. As a result of this, you will usually be asked to record your peak flows, both morning and evening, for at least one week, and often longer.

If you are used to recording your peak flows, the measurements can be particularly useful in helping you judge whether your asthma is going out of control and

Lung function tests – peak flowmeter

The most common form of lung function test is the measurement of peak expiratory flow using a peak flowmeter that measures the flow of air from your lungs. The harder you blow, the higher the reading.

Peak flowmeter
After taking a deep breath, the patient blows as hard as possible into the device. The cursor indicates the maximum speed of airflow out of the lungs.

You will usually be asked to record your peak flows both morning and evening for at least a week, on charts similar to those shown below.

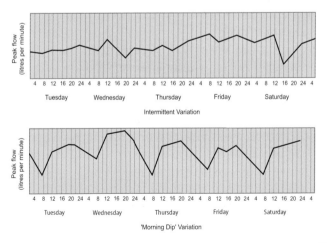

Intermittent Variation

'Morning Dip' Variation

whether you need to increase your medication. Peak flow can also be helpful in people who find it difficult to judge how bad their asthma is.

Peak flowmeters provide information that can be extremely helpful in the day-to-day management of asthma. You and your doctor can agree on a plan that allows you to judge the amount of treatment you require based on your symptoms and your peak flow readings. You can then manage change in your symptoms without having to ask for medical help every time.

Symptom diaries

Occasionally your doctor might ask you to keep a record of your symptoms on a daily basis along with details of the factors suspected of causing them. This will help you and your doctor to see the relationship between various triggers and your symptoms. As allergy often causes intermittent problems, you may be completely well on the days on which you see your doctor. A symptom diary is an accurate way of telling your doctor how frequent and how serious your symptoms are, and may give clues as to what the causes might be.

It can be quite hard work to keep a detailed symptom diary, because it may take many weeks to record sufficient details to provide the necessary information. Symptom diaries will always be subjective (you are making your own observations), but you must be as honest as possible and put down everything that you think important. Used in conjunction with a full symptom history, symptom diaries can often provide very useful clues in identifying the cause of allergic symptoms.

Trial of treatment

Sometimes allergic disease can be quite difficult to diagnose accurately, and a useful way of clinching a diagnosis is to commence appropriate anti-allergy treatment and to see whether or not your symptoms improve. This is known as a trial of treatment. Of course your doctor would weigh up the potential risks against the potential benefits and would not start any treatment unless it was safe to do so. In this situation a symptom diary (or a peak flowmeter in the case of asthma) can be extremely useful in monitoring the effect of the treatment.

Sometimes, instead of the treatment trial taking the form of a new drug or medication, a change in your environment or the avoidance of a particular allergen, for example a food, might be indicated. There are more details about allergen avoidance in the next chapter.

Tests used by alternative allergy specialists

Specialists in alternative medicine sometimes use tests that are not used in a conventional medical assessment. These tests have not been scientifically evaluated using well-conducted clinical studies. Many of them are not based on any accepted scientific theory.

Alternative therapists claim that these tests give useful information, but these claims are not backed up by any evidence and orthodox doctors are not convinced of their value. Examples are: applied kinesiology, cytotoxic testing, sublingual provocation–neutralisation, Vega testing, hair analysis and pulse tests.

Applied kinesiology

Muscle strength is measured both before and after

Example of a symptom diary

Date this card was started:			1	2	3	4

1. ASTHMA LAST NIGHT

Slept well all night..0

Awoke early, or once in night with cough or wheeze.... 1

Awoke 2–4 times.. 2

Awake for most of the night with cough or wheeze......3

2. WHEEZE AND BREATHLESSNESS TODAY

None.. 0

Mild, but not troublesome... 1

Troublesome...2

Severe...3

3. DURING EXERCISE – HOW MUCH ACTIVITY COULD YOU MANAGE TODAY?

Able to walk, run and play without cough or breathlessness..0

Normal when walking. Cough or breathlessness when running.. 1

Slight cough or breathlessness even when walking....... 2

Severe cough or breathlessness when walking. Unable to run 3

4. PEAK FLOWMETER (best of three blows standing up)   Before breakfast medicine

Before bedtime medicine

5. DRUGS	**Name of drug**	**Dose**	1	2	3	4
Number of occasions taken in past 24 hours						

5	6	7	8	9	10	11	12	13	14	15	16	17	18	19	20	21

5	6	7	8	9	10	11	12	13	14	15	16	17	18	19	20	21

exposure to a suspected allergen trigger. This test is based on the theory that allergy impairs the strength of skeletal muscle.

Cytotoxic test

This test is based on an as yet unproven theory that a food allergy alters the shape and size of white blood cells.

Sublingual provocation–neutralisation technique

In this test, increasing doses of a substance suspected of causing an allergy are administered under your tongue or as subcutaneous injections until you experience a 'sensation', thought to represent an allergic response. The nature or intensity of the symptoms or sensations is not standardised and need not be the same as the symptoms being investigated. Further concentrations of the substance are then given until you report the disappearance of symptoms.

Vega testing

This measures the electromagnetic fields that you produce both before and after you are in physical contact with an allergen.

Hair analysis

Your hair is examined and its appearance and chemical content are used to diagnose a range of medical problems.

Pulse test

A change in your pulse rate after exposure to an allergen has been claimed by some to be diagnostic of allergy to that substance. This test is usually used in cases of suspected food allergy.

None of these tests has been shown to be of any medical value.

KEY POINTS

- Accurate diagnosis of allergic problems is very important

- The results of allergy tests must be interpreted by an expert

- Skin testing is a simple, quick and inexpensive form of testing

- Patch testing is used in cases of contact dermatitis where allergy is suspected

- RAST is useful when skin-prick testing is not possible

- Peak flowmeters provide information that can be extremely helpful in the day-to-day management of asthma

- A symptom diary is an accurate way of telling your doctor how frequent and how serious your symptoms are

- Challenge tests are potentially dangerous and should never be performed at home

- Alternative or complementary medicine practitioners sometimes use tests that have not been scientifically evaluated

Treatment of allergic disease

General principles

Once allergy has been found to be the cause of your problem, the next step is to reduce your symptoms to a minimum by avoiding the allergen as far as possible and by finding an appropriate treatment. Most people with allergic problems will need to use one or more medications to control their condition. However, if you can identify the responsible allergen, it may be possible to reduce your exposure to it or to avoid it completely, and by doing so you may be able to reduce or eliminate your need for drug treatment.

Other more general measures may also help, such as maintaining good general health, eating a healthy diet, and avoiding exposure to tobacco smoke and other sources of air pollution. Finally, you may be a suitable candidate for immunotherapy (see page 110), a treatment that can damp down the allergic process, although this is not appropriate for everyone.

The aims of treatment of allergic disease are to do the following without causing excess side effects:

- reduce symptoms, particularly the frequency and severity of acute episodes
- minimise restrictions in lifestyle
- improve quality of life including the ability to enjoy work, leisure, exercise, eating, socialising and sleeping
- reduce time lost from school and work
- improve self-esteem.

Allergen avoidance

The best treatment for an allergy is to avoid completely whatever it is that triggers your symptoms, namely the allergen(s) to which you are allergic. This is relatively easy if your allergy is to something like nickel. However, there are some allergens that are impossible to avoid completely – for example, pollen and house-dust mite.

Don't despair! There are a number of practical ways in which you can reduce your contact with many allergens and in doing so minimise your need for drug treatment. We are not yet able to cure allergies but, by a combination of allergen avoidance and the right medical treatment, the symptoms of your allergy should be kept under good control.

Indoor airborne allergens

We now spend over 90 per cent of our lives indoors. Most of the air we breathe therefore comes from the indoor environment. Allergy to indoor allergens can be found in at least two out of every three patients with asthma, allergic rhinitis and eczema. The most common indoor allergens are the house-dust mite, cat dander, dog dander, pollens, moulds and spores, and, in some countries, cockroaches.

All of these allergens, combined with other factors, may make the symptoms of asthma, allergic rhinitis and eczema worse. Not only do we now spend more time inside our houses but modern houses themselves create an ideal environment for the collection of high levels of indoor allergens. Over the last 30 years houses have become warmer, with reduced levels of ventilation as a result of draught exclusion, double-glazing and the elimination of open fireplaces. As a consequence of the lack of ventilation and the higher temperatures, humidity within the home has increased. In addition, fitted carpets and soft furnishings act as reservoirs for allergens and the use of efficient detergents for clothes washing has led to the use of cooler wash temperatures that are less effective at destroying allergens that might be carried on clothing.

Another indoor environment to remember is that inside your car. We are spending increasing amounts of time in cars, and so you should make as much of an effort in keeping your car allergen free as you do with your house. Apply whatever allergen-reduction measures you are using in your house, don't let your pets on the seats if someone in the family is allergic to them, and keep it smoke free.

House-dust mite allergy

House-dust mite allergy is the most common allergy in both children and adults in the UK. House-dust mites are microscopic eight-legged insects that live on a diet of human skin scales. They grow and reproduce best in warm, humid conditions such as those found in carpets, mattresses, sofas and clothing. It is the mites' faecal (waste) particles that contain the allergen.

House dust contains large quantities of mites and their faecal particles. The house-dust mite is rare in cold countries, at high altitude and in the hospital environment.

Allergy to the house-dust mite can cause symptoms of asthma, allergic rhinitis and eczema. Before you spend a lot of time, energy and money trying to reduce the levels of house-dust mites in your home, you should first find out whether or not you are allergic to them. This can be done by skin-prick testing or by a blood test (see pages 68 and 72). If you do have a house-dust mite allergy, it is worth trying to reduce your exposure to this allergen. You can do this in the following ways.

Vacuuming
Vacuum clean regularly using a high-efficiency vacuum cleaner fitted with an efficient filter with a pore size of less than 0.3 micrometres (all manufacturers now give details of the filters that they fit). Many of the ordinary vacuum cleaners currently available meet this specification, so it is not necessary to buy an expensive 'medical' vacuum cleaner.

The information that you will need to make your choice is available from both the manufacturers and Allergy UK (see 'Useful information', page 133), which assesses many products including vacuum cleaners. If products meet their specifications, they award it their 'seal of approval'. As well as carpets, vacuum your mattress, curtains and any soft furnishings such as sofas, upholstered chairs and padded headboards (see 'Upholstery and soft furnishings' on page 133).

Beds and bedding
Beds and bedding make an ideal environment for house-

dust mites to live in. It is worth taking some protective measures to reduce your prolonged and regular exposure if you are sensitised to this allergen. There are two possible approaches here. One is to keep your bedding as allergen free as possible by regularly washing your pillows and duvet at a high temperature (at least 60°C in order to kill the house-dust mites and destroy their allergen) and by regularly vacuuming the mattress.

The other approach is to place a barrier between you and your bedding. Using barrier covers, which should completely enclose the item, is probably the easiest way to tackle your mattress, duvet and pillow. Remember to seal over the top of the zip fasteners with adhesive tape. Even if these items are full of house-dust mites, putting an efficient barrier between you and them (and their waste droppings) will prevent your symptoms being triggered.

The cheapest solution is to use plastic covers; however, these are uncomfortable because they can feel rather hot and damp and are also noisy.

More expensive anti-allergy covers are available. They are made from microporous breathable material and their cost has come down a lot in recent years. Allergy UK can provide you with details of manufacturers of items that carry the Allergy UK seal of approval. It is important to buy the whole system, including a pillow, duvet and mattress cover, otherwise the benefit will be extremely limited. As these covers are still not cheap, it is important that you confirm your house-dust mite allergy by having the appropriate tests.

Choose a bed with a slatted wood or sprung metal base. Avoid sleeping in a bed with a divan base because this makes an ideal home for the house-dust mite, and avoid sleeping on a lower bunk bed or on a

Beds and bedding

Beds and bedding make an ideal environment for house-dust mites to live in. It is worth taking some protective measures to reduce your prolonged and regular exposure if you are sensitised to this allergen.

Occlusive covers

Contained allergen

Choose a bed with a slatted wood or sprung metal base.
Use occlusive covers to seal your mattress, pillow and bedding.

Free allergen

House-dust mites live in the mattress, pillow and bedding, and so provide a regular and prolonged exposure to the allergen. A divan base reduces ventilation and provides an ideal environment for the mites to live in.

bed with a canopy because you will be under a continual shower of house-dust mite allergen.

Carpets

We spend more time in the bedroom than in any other room, so it makes sense to concentrate your efforts here. Ideally, all carpets should be removed from your bedroom and replaced with lino, vinyl, tiles or wood flooring. If you do choose to have a carpet, it is better to have a synthetic carpet because these produce a static charge that attracts the mite particles to it and so reduces the amount of allergen in the air. Vacuum the carpets and the rest of the house regularly with a high-efficiency vacuum cleaner.

Upholstery and soft furnishings

All upholstered items should be removed from your bedroom. Ideally your bedroom curtains should be unlined and made of a thin washable material. Roller blinds are a good alternative. If you can't do without them, large pieces of upholstered furniture such as divan bases and armchairs can be heat treated by a system that encloses them in a plastic cover and heats the air inside to 100°C. This treatment kills live house-dust mites and also destroys the protein of the allergen in their faecal particles (see 'Useful information', page 133).

Cuddly toys

The number of cuddly toys in the bedroom should be reduced to an absolute minimum. Any essential cuddlies should be washed regularly at a temperature of at least 60°C. Although putting these toys in the freezer will kill the living house-dust mites, it will do nothing to remove the large amount of house-dust mite allergen that can be inside, so a hot wash is preferable. If cuddly toys have to be stored in the bedroom, you should put them in a plastic box with a tightly fitting lid.

Humidity and ventilation

Increasing the ventilation of your home will reduce the humidity and so reduce the numbers of house-dust mites. The easiest and cheapest way to do this is to open the windows. A small number of air filtration systems and ionisers have been shown to lower allergen levels in the home. If you decide to buy one of these, Allergy UK (see 'Useful information', page 133) can recommend effective products.

House-dust mite sprays

There are a number of sprays available that kill house-dust mites. However, in practice these are rarely effective because the spray can penetrate only a few millimetres into furnishings. In addition, the fumes from these sprays can irritate the eyes, skin and lungs.

Pet allergens

Between 60 and 80 per cent of households in the UK have a pet of some kind – cats are the most popular. At least a third of people with allergies are allergic to pet allergens – so these are a major trigger factor in allergic disease.

It is not necessary to handle an animal to come into contact with its allergen. The allergen can travel in small particles in the air and can be passed from person to person or from house to house on clothing and footwear. The allergen can be found in the fur and skin scales, saliva, urine and faeces of the animal.

No matter where in the home the pet lives, the allergen will quickly become distributed around the rest of the house, and so it is not enough to restrict the pet to certain parts of the home in the hope that the other rooms will remain allergen free. Animal allergens persist for a long time and, once a pet has left a home, it may take many months of hard work with an efficient vacuum cleaner to remove most of the allergen.

If you are allergic to pet allergen, the obvious answer is not to keep that pet. However, we are a nation of animal lovers and some families are very reluctant to let their pet go. If you decide that you want to keep a pet that makes your symptoms worse, try to keep your contact with the animal to a minimum. Maybe it can live outside or in the garage and never come into the house. When you or another family member strokes or handles the animal you should wear special clothing which you do not bring into the house. Leave the clothing in the garage or put it straight into the washing machine. Use a high-efficiency vacuum cleaner regularly to remove as much of the allergen as possible from the home.

Consider washing your cat regularly – although this is easier said than done! Studies have shown that washing a cat once a week, particularly if you ask your vet for a special shampoo, significantly reduces the amount of allergen that it sheds.

Pollen

Plants can be pollinated in two ways: by insects and wind. It is the wind-pollinated plants that cause trouble for the sufferer of seasonal allergic rhinitis (hay fever). These plants produce huge quantities of pollen because wind pollination is not very efficient. The particles can

Generalised pollen calendar for the UK

This calendar shows the general pattern of pollen release in the UK. The exact timing and severity of pollen seasons will vary from year to year depending on the weather, and also regionally depending on geographical location.

Plant (genus)	Jan	Feb	Mar	Apr	May	Jun	Jul	Aug	Sep
Hazel (*Corylus*)	■	●■	■						
Yew (*Taxus*)		●■	■						
Elm (*Ulmus*)		■	●■	■					
Alder (*Alnus*)	■	■	●■	■					
Willow (*Salix*)			●■	■	■				
Ash (*Fraxinus*)			■	●■	■				
Poplar (*Populus*)			●■	■					
Birch (*Betula*)			■	●■	■				
Oak (*Quercus*)				■	●■	■			
Pine (*Pinus*)				■	●■	■			
Grass (*Gramineae*)					■	●■	●■	■	
Oil seed Rape (*Brassica napus*)				■	●■	■			
Plane (*Platanus*)			■	●■	■	■			
Dock (*Rumex*)					■	●■	■	■	
Nettle (*Urtica*)					■	●■	●■	■	■
Lime (*Tilia*)						●■	■		
Plantain (*Plantago*)					■	●■	■	■	
Mugwort (*Artemisia*)							●■	●■	

Key: ● Peak period of pollen release ■ Pollen season

Information supplied by the National Pollen Research Unit, University College, Worcester.

Generalised pollen variation over the day

The graph below shows the generalised variation in the amount of grass pollen in the air at times measured over the period of a day in the UK on warm days during the season of peak release (June and early July).

Information supplied by the National Pollen Research Unit, University College, Worcester.

be carried for long distances, because they are small and dry and therefore light. So, although this type of pollen is very difficult to avoid, there are useful things that you can do:

- Identify which pollens cause your allergies by skin-prick testing. You can then find out when to expect trouble from these pollens because each plant flowers at a predictable time each year. Once you know this, you should start your hay fever treatments at least two weeks before the time your symptoms would usually start. This will decrease the intensity of your symptoms and reduce the amount of medications that you take overall.

- Spend as little time out of doors as possible during the pollen season, especially when the pollen count is high. The pollen count will rise on warm, dry, sunny days.

- Try to do your outdoor activities at a time that the pollen count is likely to be lower, for example, early morning or any time after rainfall, which will reduce the pollen count.

- Check the pollen count using the internet or local newspapers when planning outdoor activities.

- Wear glasses when out of doors, because this will give your eyes some protection from the pollen.

- Change your clothes when you come indoors if the pollen count has been high.

- Do not dry your clothes and bed linen out of doors in summer, because they will become covered in pollen.

- Keep your bedroom window closed during the pollen season.

- If you can, arrange your holiday during your worst time of year and go to a country where your trigger pollen is not found. Otherwise, go to the seaside where inshore sea breezes keep the pollen count low.

- If you are allergic to grass pollen, do not cut the grass yourself.

- Some cars now have efficient air filters that trap pollen and make the interior relatively pollen free. Consider choosing one when you next change your car.

- Do your gardening on cold, wet or dull days.

- Choose plants that are insect pollinated, because the pollen from these is much heavier and less likely to cause symptoms.

- Control weeds in the garden, because many of these produce troublesome pollens.

- Do not have fresh flowers in the house/office/classroom during your hay fever season – they may be from plants to which you are allergic.

- Avoid things that will make your symptoms worse – such as exposure to smoke, fumes and other forms of air pollution.

Food allergens

Once you have been diagnosed as having an allergy to one or more foodstuffs, face up to your allergy, don't just hope it will go away. None of the preventive allergy drugs works in food allergy, nor does immunotherapy, so the most effective management is to avoid completely the allergen in question (food elimination). You must not eliminate too many food types from your diet at once, otherwise your diet might become deficient in certain essential nutrients and you still won't know which food is the problem. In the case of growing children, no food should be eliminated long term without medical and dietetic advice.

It is possible to grow out of a food allergy. If you have been free of allergic reactions for several years, your doctor can arrange allergy tests. If these are negative, he or she can then arrange a controlled challenge test, which MUST be performed in a safe hospital setting.

It is important that you do not eliminate foods from your diet unless you have a proven allergy. Many people wrongly blame food allergy for a wide range of symptoms and because of this they limit their choice of food, and therefore their lifestyle, for no real benefit. They may even become malnourished.

Eliminating any foodstuff completely from your diet can be difficult, because it is not always easy to know all the ingredients of packaged and pre-prepared foods. You will need to read food labels very carefully and to learn the different names by which different foodstuffs can be identified. You should read the labels each time you buy a food, as manufacturers sometimes change the ingredients without notice.

All the major supermarket chains provide 'free-from' lists, indicating, for example, which foods do not contain egg (see 'Useful information', page 133). These are updated regularly and can be very helpful, especially when buying pre-prepared foods. A dietitian can give you helpful advice on 'hidden' sources of different foods.

Milk

Milk is found in many foods as well as in the form of a drink. Words used to describe milk include whey, casein, caseinates, lactose, dry milk solids and milk powder. Casein is used in some non-dairy foods as a binder, and may be found in canned tuna and in some meats. You must avoid butter, cheese, cream, yoghurt, crème fraiche, fromage frais, condensed milk, evaporated milk, ice cream and milk chocolate – and any food that lists any of these as ingredients. Margarines and spreads sometimes contain butter. Goats' milk is not a safe alternative to cows' milk because it contains a very similar protein. Lactose, a milk sugar, is often used in pharmaceutical preparations and tablets, so read the patient information leaflets of all medications that you are prescribed. Beware the restaurant practice of putting butter on vegetables and steaks after they are cooked – once it has melted it is difficult to see.

Eggs

Egg is found in a wide variety of processed foods. It is important to read the contents list carefully – it may be described by a number of names, including albumin, egg white and dried egg. Eggs are often used as glazing on baked goods.

Peanut

Peanut can also be labelled as *arachis* or *groundnut*. The peanut allergen is not destroyed by cooking. Beware peanut/groundnut oil, because, although most are made by distillation and these oils do not contain any protein and so are allergen free, cold-pressed oils can contain dangerous amounts of allergen. Avoid all assorted selections of chocolate sweets because usually at least one type contains peanut and the others can be contaminated at some stage during the manufacturing process. Peanuts are cheap, and are often deflavoured and then reflavoured as a tree nut, so it is best to avoid all tree nut products too. It is almost impossible to guarantee that bakery and ice-cream items have not been contaminated by peanut. If your child has a peanut allergy, make sure that he never swaps food with other children, for example at school.

Sesame

Hummus, tahini and halvah are three popular sesame products. Sesame seeds in other food products can generally be identified from the labels. However, it is possible that products labelled as containing 'vegetable oil' may contain sesame.

Some foodstuffs are chemically related to others and so, if you develop an allergy to one, you may also react to another. This is called cross-reactivity. For example, celery, apple, peanuts and kiwi fruit are all related and their common allergen has been identified. Similarly, bananas, kiwi fruit, papaya, chestnuts and avocados appear to be related, and allergies to all of these can occur in patients who are allergic to latex.

Even small amounts of allergen can be dangerous. If your child is allergic to peanuts, for example, even sitting next to another child eating peanut butter sandwiches can cause a reaction when small particles become airborne. Ask the school if they might make the classroom/dining hall peanut free. Most headteachers will be very understanding.

If you have a severe food allergy, develop a treatment plan. Make sure that your friends, work colleagues or schoolteachers, and family know what your symptoms are, where to find your drugs and how to administer them.

When you are eating out, avoid high-risk restaurants, such as those serving Indian and Eastern dishes, which include a wide range of different ingredients that can be difficult to identify, and in which nuts and peanuts are commonly used. Even if the dish that you order does not contain your allergen, the pan in which it is cooked may have been previously been used to cook one that does.

Be direct with the restaurant staff, and ask to speak in person to the chef if you think that the waiter is not taking you seriously. Share your problem with your friends so that they can help you in choosing appropriate food, and teach them about your symptoms and how to treat them.

Be alert and do not ignore any symptom, however mild. It could be the start of a serious reaction. Finally, if you have been prescribed epinephrine, always carry it with you when you go out, and use it if you even suspect that you might be having a reaction. It is better to risk the mild embarrassment when no reaction occurs than to ignore the early signs of a serious allergic reaction and not receive the help that you need in time.

Management of food allergy

- Don't eliminate any food from your diet until an allergy to it has been accurately diagnosed

- Get help from a dietitian

- Learn the different names used for your food allergen

- Read the ingredients lists on packaged foods carefully – manufacturers may change the contents without warning

- Don't rely on kosher labelling of milk-free foods – they might still contain a trace of milk

- Use supermarket 'free-from' lists

- Be aware of the possibility of cross-reactivity with other foods

- For children, enlist the help and cooperation of other mothers and the school staff

- Teach your child how to decipher food labels and other strategies for avoiding problem foods

- Consider taking your own food when eating at other people's homes

- Choose your restaurants carefully and avoid Asian food because the individual ingredients can be difficult to identify and many Asian cuisines use peanuts quite heavily

- Develop a relationship with the chef or owner of your favourite restaurant

- Take even mild symptoms seriously
- Wear a medical identification bracelet (see page 60)
- If you have been prescribed epinephrine, carry your injectors with you at all times.

Stinging insects

Most people develop a painful and itchy skin weal if stung by a bee or a wasp. This is normal, and not an allergic reaction. However, some people become sensitised to a protein in the venom, and are then at risk of an allergic reaction, which can be severe. There are many things that you can do to reduce the chances of your being stung by a wasp or bee:

- Use an effective insect repellent when spending time outdoors.
- Wear plain, light-coloured clothes and avoid brightly coloured flower prints and black – these seem to attract insects.
- Never disturb wasp nests or beehives.
- If you discover an insect nest, call the council or a company such as Rentokil to deal with it.
- Do not walk barefoot out of doors.
- Avoid wearing strong perfumes and any cosmetic preparations with a strong fragrance.
- Keep your arms and legs covered.
- Stay away from picnic grounds and the areas around dustbins and litterbins – wasps are particularly attracted by rubbish.
- Keep patios, dustbin areas and barbecues clean.
- Get someone else to mow the lawn.

- Deal with any pools of water that collect in your garden – insects are attracted by them.
- Don't drink directly from cans of fizzy drink – an insect could have flown in and you won't be able to see it.
- Make sure that no bees or wasps are inside your car before you get in.
- If a bee or wasp comes near you, do not attack it, but move slowly and calmly away.
- If an insect lands on you, try to stay calm and leave it alone until it flies away – it will not sting you unless it feels threatened.

Drug treatments

It is not possible to avoid all relevant allergens all of the time so, although allergen avoidance should play an important part in the management of your allergies, this approach may need to be combined with the use of appropriate anti-allergy drugs. There are five main groups of drugs:

1 Symptomatic relievers – taken for immediate relief of the symptoms.

2 Antihistamines – which reduce the severity of the allergic reaction by blocking the effects of histamine once it has been released by the inflammatory cells.

3 Anti-inflammatories – which reduce the levels of inflammation by preventing the release of the chemicals, including histamine.

4 Leukotriene receptor antagonists – a newer class of drug developed specifically for use in allergic diseases. These drugs block the receptor to which leukotrienes (one type of inflammatory chemical) have to attach before they can cause inflammation.

This prevents that part of the immune reaction from occurring.

5 Immune-modulating agents – a new class of skin treatment for atopic dermatitis.

In addition, epinephrine is used for the treatment of acute/severe allergic reactions (see page 109).

It is important to remember that all allergic conditions change over time, and that you and your doctor must continually re-evaluate your treatment requirements. Your aim should be to get the maximum possible benefit from the lowest possible dose of medication.

Provided that you are able to communicate clearly and frequently with your doctor, and avoid the trap of having low expectations of your quality of life, together you will be able to fine-tune your treatment to achieve the best possible control.

Symptomatic relievers

These drugs should be used to treat your symptoms at the time you are experiencing a flare-up.

The lungs

Every person with asthma should carry with them a 'reliever' inhaler, containing a drug that relaxes the airway muscle and dilates the small airways or bronchi (a bronchodilator). It should be in a form that the person finds easy to use even when breathless and wheezy.

There is one situation in which your reliever inhaler can be used to *prevent* symptoms – if used 15 minutes before exercise, it will prevent you from developing exercise-induced wheeze and cough.

The eyes

A range of eye drops is available that will temporarily reduce the redness, crying and stinging associated with hay fever. These drops contain drugs that constrict the blood vessels on the surface of the eye. However, these drops should not be used for prolonged periods of more than one week. Long-term use will make your condition worse because, when the effects of each dose wear off, your symptoms will reappear worse than before – rebound symptoms. They should also be avoided in people with glaucoma (raised pressure inside the eye), high blood pressure and diabetes.

The nose

Decongestant nose drops or sprays work in the same way as decongestant eye drops, by constricting the blood vessels in the lining of the nose. This leads to a decrease in nasal secretions and relief of nasal obstruction.

Although these drugs work rapidly and can be very effective, they should not be used in the long term because they can lead to a worsening of your symptoms. It is far better to protect yourself from your allergic symptoms rather than to treat the end result. You should seek treatment with anti-inflammatories to reduce your inflammatory response and also avoid the allergen as much as possible.

The skin

Inflamed skin can be very itchy and the regular use of simple emollient creams will not only relieve the itching but also make your skin stronger. These creams do not contain any drugs, but act to smooth the surface of the skin and to increase its degree of hydration by reducing

> **Helpful tip**
>
> If your skin is feeling really itchy, instead of scratching, which will make the itch worse, take a generous handful of emollient cream and rub it gently but firmly into the itchy areas

water loss. Both of these actions strengthen your skin by making it thicker and less rough. The creams that your doctor can prescribe for you (some are also available to buy from pharmacies) are more effective than cosmetic moisturiser creams and are less likely to irritate your skin because they contain no perfumes and most are lanolin free.

There are other things that you can do to help:

- Wearing clothes made of cotton next to your skin helps prevent itching and scratching
- If you are allergic to the house-dust mite, use barrier covers on your mattress, duvet and pillow, and avoid divan bases (see page 87)
- Moisturise the skin regularly, several times a day
- Keep fingernails short – if you scratch you will damage your skin less
- Be alert for signs of skin infection – this may need treatment with antibiotics.

Antihistamines

Antihistamine drugs act by reducing the ability of histamine to attach to the cell receptors where it exerts its effect. Histamine is one of the most potent inflammatory chemicals released by the body during the inflammatory reaction. Histamine can cause airway narrowing, abdominal cramps, sneezing, and itching and watering of the nose and eyes. Antihistamine medications can be supplied as eye drops, nasal sprays, and tablets or liquid preparations to take by mouth. Sometimes an antihistamine preparation alone will be enough to prevent your symptoms.

However, they are not very good at treating a blocked congested nose caused by hay fever and, for this, an anti-inflammatory preparation (see below) will be needed.

The most common side effect of antihistamines is sedation (drowsiness), and the effect of some of the older antihistamines on your ability to drive may be as serious as the effects of alcohol. These drugs are still used at night in severe cases of allergy when their sedative effect can be useful in promoting sleep. Chlorpheniramine (Piriton) has probably the greatest sedating effect. It may be useful when you are finding it hard to sleep at night because of your symptoms, but should not be used during the day if you will be driving, cooking or operating machinery. However, because it works quickly, it is the antihistamine of choice for treatment of an acute severe allergic reaction. Some of the new or second-generation drugs are non-sedating – for example, loratadine, acrivastine and astemizole. They are easier to take too, because they are taken only once, or at most twice, a day.

Anti-inflammatory drugs

Anti-inflammatory medications suppress inflammation and so reduce the changes in the tissues and lessen or even eliminate symptoms. In order to do their job, these medications must be taken regularly, and they work

Allergic rhinitis (hayfever): which treatment is best?

	Sneezing/ itch	Watery discharge	Blocked nose	Eye symptoms
Sodium cromoglycate	+	+	−	+
Antihistamines	+++	++	−	+++
Nasal steroids	+++	+++	++	+
Decongestants	−	−	+++	−

− No effect, + limited effectiveness, + + quite effective, + + + very effective

better with fewer side effects if applied locally to the affected part of the body. It may take several weeks for their effect to become noticeable.

There are two main classes of anti-inflammatory drugs.

Sodium cromoglycate and nedocromil
These preparations are available as eye drops, nasal sprays, asthma inhalers and for taking by mouth (oral preparations) – although this form is rarely used. It is worth trying these drugs if your symptoms are mild, because they have no side effects whatsoever. However, they are not particularly potent preparations and may have limited efficacy.

Corticosteroids
The corticosteroid group of drugs is the most useful and effective for the treatment of allergic conditions. They are available in a full range of preparations including skin creams, eye drops, nasal sprays and

asthma inhalers, as well as oral preparations, which are used for the treatment of severe or acute symptoms.

Many patients are concerned about using corticosteroid preparations, because they are frightened about possible side effects. First, it is important to understand that corticosteroid medications are not the same as the anabolic steroids sometimes used and abused by body builders and athletes.

Second, corticosteroids are usually given topically (locally onto the part of the body that needs treatment), for example, by inhalation for asthma and as creams for eczema. As a result of this, the doses used can be very small, and side effects are minimised. It is only in high doses and if taken over a prolonged period that cortico-steroids will lead to side effects, which may include:

- thin skin
- easy bruising
- thinning of the bones (osteoporosis)
- underactivity of the adrenal gland – leading to collapse in severe cases
- growth suppression in children.

By using topical preparations, for example an inhaler or a nasal spray, you will be taking a dose of cortico-steroid only one-fiftieth or one-hundredth of the dose you would have to take orally to get the same effect, and you are very unlikely to develop side effects.

Unless you have very severe asthma, you will not need to take regular oral steroid preparations. Using oral steroids for a number of days when you have an acute severe attack of your asthma is unlikely to have any undesirable effects. Beware, however, if you are using high doses of a steroid inhaler, nose spray or skin cream, or if you are using a combination of these different treatments, because their ability to cause side effects is additive and on a high enough dose serious side effects are possible.

If you are taking high doses of any one steroid medication or if you are taking a combination of different steroid medications, you should bring this to the attention of your doctor. He or she will try to reduce the doses that you use to the minimum that still provides good treatment of your symptoms. If children are on high doses of steroid treatments, they should be re-evaluated regularly and the doses reduced wherever possible. In addition, their growth should be carefully monitored.

Leukotriene receptor antagonists

A relatively new class of drug has become available for the treatment of asthma – the leukotriene receptor antagonists (LRAs). These drugs can also be very effective in the treatment of allergic rhinitis and eczema. The two drugs currently available are montelukast and zafirlukast.

For many patients, the best thing about these drugs is that they are taken by mouth in tablet form. These drugs are usually prescribed for people with asthma that is severe enough for them to be already taking a steroid inhaler. After a period of treatment you may be able to reduce the dose of your steroid inhaler. If you also have hay fever and eczema, these are likely to improve.

The most common side effect of these drugs is headache, which tends to disappear if you persevere with treatment for a couple of weeks.

Unfortunately, these drugs are not effective in everyone – some people respond well and others not at all. When your doctor starts you on one of these medications, he will probably ask you to keep a record of your symptoms for three to four weeks so that you can both see whether or not you are benefiting.

Immune-modulating agents

Until recently there was only one class of medication used in skin creams for atopic dermatitis, and this was the corticosteroids. There is a new family of drugs, for use topically, that appear to have many of the benefits of steroid creams without many of the disadvantages. Two of these, tacrolimus (Protopic) and pimecrolimus (Elidel), are currently available as skin creams. They are related to a drug, ciclosporin, that is used as an immunosuppressant in organ transplantation.

These are for use in patients whose eczema has not responded to conventional treatments and, although they do have significant side effects of their own and so are generally prescribed by specialists, the results so far are promising. However, their long-term safety and place in therapy are still being evaluated.

Epinephrine

Epinephrine (adrenaline) is a chemical that occurs naturally in the body, produced by the adrenal gland. Epinephrine has a number of actions, including relaxation of the airways and reversal of the leakiness of the small blood vessels, which may be helpful in the event of a severe allergic reaction.

Epinephrine must be given by injection, usually into a muscle, although in hospital it might be injected directly into a vein. It can be supplied in kits that are easy to use by the patient him- or herself (see 'Anaphylaxis', page 56).

The most popular device, the EpiPen, looks like a pen and can easily be carried with you at all times. Epinephrine works quickly but its effects may wear off after approximately 30 minutes whereas an allergic reaction can continue for many hours. As a result of this, you may require a second dose to buy you enough time to reach medical attention. For this reason, you should always carry two devices, and once you have injected epinephrine you should immediately dial 999 and get medical help.

Immunotherapy

Immunotherapy, also known as desensitisation, is a process by which a patient is rendered less sensitive to an allergen. This is done by giving the patient increasing doses of the substance to which he or she is allergic, starting with extremely small quantities. The allergen is usually given by injection, but can also be delivered into the mouth or nose.

If this treatment is successful, the numbers of basophils and mast cells are reduced, their sensitivity to allergen is reduced, and the levels of allergen-specific IgE are lowered. However, you need to be really committed to this therapy because it requires frequent treatments over several years, and the risk of an acute severe allergic reaction is considerable.

Immunotherapy should be used only in patients who have an allergy resulting in severe symptoms that cannot be controlled by conventional drug therapy combined with allergen avoidance. It works best in people who are allergic to only one allergen, although it may work in multiple allergies.

The most common conditions treated by immuno-therapy include hay fever caused by pollen and severe allergy to bee and wasp stings. Immunotherapy is rarely used for the treatment of asthma. Only one allergen should be treated at any time.

In the UK, a relatively small number of people are treated with immunotherapy because of the onerous treatment period and the risk of serious allergic reactions (see below). As a result of this risk, it must be carried out only in specialist allergy centres.

Immunotherapy injections

These are given under the skin (subcutaneously) each week or even twice a week, starting with minute doses. Increasing concentrations of the allergen are used over several months until the highest planned dose is reached. That dose is then repeated once a month to maintain the benefit. The whole course can last several years.

The advantages of this treatment are that in carefully chosen patients this can be a very effective form of therapy and, after completion of the course, the benefits can be long lasting.

The disadvantages are as follows:

- The treatment is time-consuming, because you will need to remain under observation for several hours after each dose and many doses are given, initially as often as twice a week.

- The duration of the course is long, being several years, so it is a major commitment.

- Approximately half of patients suffer a relapse of their symptoms, usually after two to three years.

This treatment can have dangerous side effects. You are being exposed to the allergen responsible for your symptoms, so there is a risk of a severe allergic reaction. This risk is greatest in patients who also have asthma, especially if their asthma is not under good control. Between three and twelve per cent of patients suffer a severe allergic reaction, most but not all of these occurring within 30 minutes of the injection. This is why you are required to remain at the hospital for several hours after each injection.

Very rarely, the allergic reaction can be so severe that it is fatal. For this reason, the selection of patients to receive immunotherapy is made very carefully, and the procedure is carried out only by specialists working in specialist hospital centres.

Oral and nasal immunotherapy

In an attempt to reduce the risks of immunotherapy, other routes for giving the doses of allergen have been tried. The oral and nasal routes require higher doses of allergen, are slower to work and carry a greater risk of causing urticaria and angio-oedema. However, the risk of anaphylaxis is lower than with the subcutaneous injections.

Unfortunately, these routes are less effective and the results not as good as with injections. The nasal route seems to provide benefit locally in the nose only, so it is effective only for allergic rhinitis.

What else can I do?

Your symptoms should be well controlled if your allergies have been diagnosed correctly, if you have reduced your exposure to the relevant allergen adequately and if you are taking appropriate medication. However, there are other things that you can do to help.

Irritants

If you can avoid exposure to substances likely to act as irritants, you will be less vulnerable to the effects of your allergies.

A wide range of substances can cause irritant reactions in your lungs, nose, eyes and skin, and the most common of these is tobacco smoke. If you currently smoke you should try to give up. If you are a non-smoker, you should reduce as much as possible your exposure to other people's cigarette smoke. Babies and small children should never be allowed to breathe in cigarette smoke.

Raised levels of air pollutants – for example, car exhaust fumes, ozone, formaldehyde and nitrous oxide – can also make your allergy symptoms worse. As we spend most of our time indoors, it makes sense to keep our home environment as free as possible from smoke and fumes. Keep your house well ventilated, especially the rooms that contain a gas burner or pilot light of any kind. At work, make sure that your employer protects you from inhaling any dusts or fumes. Outdoors, avoid, if you can, walking along busy roads where you will be exposed to high levels of car exhaust fumes and dust.

Identification jewellery

If someone in your family has a severe allergy, you may find it reassuring to obtain a piece of medical identification jewellery for them which carries details of their medical problem as well as their personal details and their doctor's name and telephone number. These can be provided by a number of different companies, each of which offers a different service. Details of how to contact MedicAlert, SOS Talisman and Golden Key can be found under 'Useful information' (page 133). MedicAlert, a charity established in 1965, maintains an up-to-date computerised database of its members' medical conditions and they make this available to the emergency services.

Complementary therapies

There is a wide range of different treatments offered by a variety of practitioners. I think it is important to draw the distinction between *alternative* therapies, which aim to replace the treatments offered by the medical profession, and *complementary* therapies, which are intended for use alongside conventional treatments.

As the effects of severe allergy can be very unpleasant and even life threatening, it is important that you do not suddenly stop the medications prescribed for you by your doctor. If an alternative therapist tells you that his or her treatments will not work unless you give up your other medications, speak to your doctor first. In my opinion, these other therapies work best when used in conjunction with conventional medicine.

Very little is known about how complementary therapies work, but, if you find one that works for you and you can afford the treatment, then I would encourage you to use it. However, complementary therapies should never be relied on in the case of a sudden acute allergic reaction, when conventional medicines will offer you the most effective solutions.

It is worth bearing in mind that many complementary therapists have no formal medical training and might not have the experience or the knowledge to diagnose and treat your medical problems properly. Other diseases can sometimes mimic the symptoms of allergy, and may be misdiagnosed by complementary therapists.

Complementary therapies are often regarded as a low-risk option, but dangerous side effects can occur and, at worst, they could actually kill you. The Chinese herbal medicine *Aristolochia* has caused kidney failure in a number of patients and was banned in 1999. In 1998,

Questions to ask your complementary therapist

- What training have you had?
- What are your qualifications?
- How much experience do you have?
- Are you registered with a recognised organisation?
- What will the treatment involve?
- Is this the best treatment for me?
- What benefits can I expect?
- Will you tell my GP about this treatment?
- Are you happy for me to continue my normal medications?
- How many sessions do you recommend?
- How much will this cost?

12 patients contracted hepatitis B, which is potentially fatal, in London from a therapy called autohaemotherapy.

In the UK there are 40,000 complementary therapists and they now outnumber registered GPs (31,000). Yet complementary therapists are largely unregulated, and registration with a professional body is not compulsory.

If you are thinking of seeking help from a complementary therapist, it is worth ensuring that he or she is suitably qualified and regulated. You can contact the Department of Health (see 'Useful information', page 133) and ask if they will give you the names of recommended practitioners in your area. Your GP might be able to help you with this. You can also contact the relevant professional body, such as the British Acupuncture Council (see 'Useful information', page 133). See also *Understanding Complementary Medicine*, another book in the Family Doctor series.

Brief guide to complementary medicine
Acupuncture

Acupuncture is an ancient Chinese medical practice. Diagnosis is based on an assessment of the patient's mood, character and life situation. Treatment aims to improve the flow of energy through clearly defined channels in the body, clearing blockages to this flow that result in illness.

This is done by the insertion of very fine steel needles into specific points along the channels of energy flow.

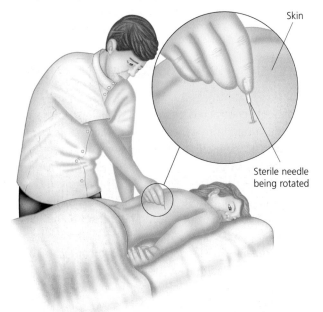

Skin

Sterile needle being rotated

Acupuncture is a method of pain relief that involves insertion of fine sterile needles into specific points on the body. The needles may then be rotated to produce stimulation.

The needles are left in place for between 5 and 30 minutes. Although acupuncture is sometimes recommended for asthma and hay fever, the treatments need to be very frequent and, as yet, there is no scientific proof that it offers any benefit for these conditions.

Homeopathy

The practice of homeopathy is based on the theory that 'like cures like'. Minute quantities of the substance believed to mimic the symptoms of disease are given to treat that disease. The remedies are taken by mouth.

The results of homeopathy can be slow and initially symptoms may become worse. However, the remedies are felt to be safe because they contain such tiny quantities of the substance used. Although homeopathy

Dr Samuel Hahnemann (1755–1843), German physician and pioneer of homeopathy.

is recommended for the treatment of all allergic diseases by its practitioners, it is only in hay fever that homeopathy seems to offer a benefit detectable by scientific studies.

Enzyme-potentiated desensitisation

In this treatment a very small dose of the allergen or a number of different relevant allergens is mixed with an enzyme (beta-glucuronidase) and the mixture injected under the skin. A single dose is said to give lasting benefit, and its supporters believe that it is effective in many different allergic diseases.

However, at the moment there is very little evidence to prove this and more studies are needed. Severe adverse reactions to this treatment can occur and it should be performed only in a place, for example a specialised allergy clinic or a sizeable hospital, where such reactions can be quickly and properly treated and resuscitation given if needed.

Herbal medicine

Herbal medicines made from the leaves, flowers, bark or roots of plants have been used for thousands of years. In some parts of the world it is the only form of medicine used. Western herbalists prescribe a combination of different herbal remedies specific to an individual's problem. In addition, Chinese herbal therapies have gained in popularity and have been found to be very effective in eczema. However, some products have been found to be contaminated or augmented with other substances such as steroid preparations, and others have led to serious complications such as liver damage. Only seek treatment from a reputable therapist (see 'Useful information', page 133).

Herbal
infusion

Strainer

Herbal tea

Herbal medicine involves the use of plant extracts to treat illness. The remedy is often prepared as a 'tea' to drink.

KEY POINTS

- We cannot yet cure allergies

- Most people's symptoms can be well controlled using a combination of allergen avoidance and drug treatment

- Whatever the allergen to which you are allergic, there are many practical ways in which you can reduce your exposure to it

- The most common allergy in the UK is to the house-dust mite

- The indoor environment is the most relevant to your allergy as we spend about 90 per cent of our time indoors

- Learn all about your drug treatment, including how and when to use it, so that you may use it effectively

- Immunotherapy is used only in people whose allergy symptoms are severe and in whom drug treatment and allergen avoidance are not effective

- A wide range of complementary therapies is available

- Choose your complementary therapist with care

Living with allergies

School

If your child has an allergic condition, you may be anxious about how well the school is able to cope. It may help to remember that as many as a third of the children in the school will have some type of allergic condition and the teachers will have considerable experience in dealing with all the related problems. However, it is only sensible to make sure that the school has all the information that may be relevant to your child and his or her medical problem. Make sure that you include the following information:

- The condition your child has
- The things to which your child is allergic
- The names and doses of all the medications that your child takes regularly
- The names and doses of the medications that your child will need to take at school on a regular basis.
- How to recognise when your child is having an allergic reaction
- The names and doses of the medications that your child might need to take in the event of an allergic reaction

- A treatment plan of exactly what to do if your child develops an allergic reaction
- Details of the triggers known to make your child's condition worse
- The name and telephone number of your general practitioner
- Telephone numbers where you, your partner and other nominated adults can be contacted in an emergency.

Every school receives instructions from the Department for Education and Skills (DfES), in conjunction with the local education authority, on putting an asthma policy in place, covering details such as the storage and administration of children's asthma inhalers in school. If your child has other allergies, you might find it helpful to give the school relevant information such as that produced by Allergy UK or the Anaphylaxis Campaign (see 'Useful information', page 133).

If your child has a severe allergic problem, it is important to spend some time with the relevant members of staff to discuss your child's needs. In the UK, all children, including those with special medical needs, have a right to full education in state schools, and their teachers must, within reason, take responsibility for the child's medical needs while they are at school. The DfES and the Department of Health have issued joint guidelines on supporting pupils with medical needs in school. Copies can be obtained from the DfES (see 'Useful information', page 133).

Food

Food in school can be an issue for children with food allergies. It should still be possible for children with food allergies to eat school meals, but they will need special supervision by a member of staff to ensure that they make appropriate choices. It may be easier to provide your child with a packed lunch. Many schools now have a no-sharing policy to ensure that children eat only the food provided for them. Some schools are willing to make certain areas free from certain allergens, for example peanuts. Make sure that your child will have access to their medications at all times in case they accidentally eat the wrong food.

Exercise and sport

Exercise and sport can present difficulties to many children with allergic problems. Exercise can make asthma worse. Outdoor sports may expose children to high levels of pollen that could make asthma, hay fever or eczema worse. Although swimming is a form of exercise well tolerated by children with asthma, it can make eczema much worse. There are ways of getting round these problems (see 'Useful information', page 133) so that all children are able to join in with all school activities including sport.

Hay fever

Some parents worry that their child's hay fever may affect their performance in examinations, which generally take place during the pollen season. The following may be helpful:

- Start appropriate preventive medications several weeks before the hay fever season commences. It is harder to gain control of symptoms once they have started than it is to prevent them.

- Your child may need to use more than one medication. Often the combination of an antihistamine, a nasal spay and eye drops works best.

- Make sure that your child takes medications regularly.

- Follow the advice on pollen avoidance (see 'Treatment of allergic disease', page 83).

- If your child is sitting examinations and is troubled by hay fever, ask the school or college to inform the examining board.

Holidays and travel

Some people, especially those with severe allergic problems, never go away on holiday because of their fear of what may happen in an unknown environment. It is a great shame because, with the right information and some forward planning, a holiday can be a very enjoyable experience regardless of the allergy.

It is possible to remove or at least minimise many potential hazards by maintaining control over the important aspects of your life while you are on holiday. For example, if you have a severe food allergy, you could choose to stay in self-catering accommodation. If you have hay fever, you might choose to visit the southern hemisphere where not only will the season differ from that at home but also the local pollens will differ.

Alternatively you might consider a seaside holiday because the pollen count is generally lower on the coast. If you have asthma, you may be able to take appropriate rescue medications with you so that, with careful instructions from your doctor, you could treat any exacerbation early.

Do remember to take sufficient supplies of your medication with you to last throughout the holiday,

General advice for parents of children with allergies

Remember the following:

- Make sure that your child takes his or her preventive medications regularly.

- Make sure that children have access to their reliever medications at all times while in school.

- If your child has asthma and exercise is a problem, advise taking two puffs of their reliever inhaler at least 15 minutes before exercise.

- If your child has eczema, make sure that she or he wears natural fibres (for example, cotton) next to the skin and avoid wool, which can irritate the skin.

- If your child has eczema, make sure that she or he can shower thoroughly after swimming to remove the chemicals and, if needed, re-apply their emollient cream.

- If your child has a food allergy, make sure that the school is well informed of this. Ensure that the school dining room has a no-sharing policy. Ask the school to warn you in advance of what ingredients will be used in domestic science (cookery) lessons and ask whether the relevant food stuffs might be avoided.

- Find out whether the school has any pets or other animals on the premises. If they do and your child is allergic to them, ask if you may visit the school to discuss how your child might avoid exposure to the allergen.

- If your child has a **severe** food allergy, make sure that the school and the child's classmates are well aware of this, and request that all of the children be made to wash their hands and faces thoroughly after eating so that food allergens are not spread around by touch after meals.

and always carry your medications in your hand luggage just in case your main luggage goes astray. Other points to remember are:

- Choose a destination that in your experience is least likely to trigger your allergy.

- If you have any special requirements, such as a special diet or feather-free bedding, ask your holiday company well in advance to supply these and ask for confirmation in writing.

- Make sure that you have adequate medical insurance and do tell your insurer about your medical problem.

- If you are going to a European Union country, take your European Health Insurance Card (EHIC), available from any post office – you can use it to get free or subsidised medical care. If you do not have an EHIC, details of how to apply for one can be found on the Department of Health website (see 'Useful information', page 133) or are available from any post office. The EHIC supersedes form E111, which is invalid from 1 January 2006.

- Take with you a written action plan covering what you would do if you have an exacerbation while on holiday.

- Check the expiry dates of your medications.

- If you have been prescribed an epinephrine device, take extra supplies with you in case you need to use them more than once. It will be difficult to organise replacements abroad.

- Protect your epinephrine device from extremes of temperature (don't leave it in the car), and discard it if the epinephrine becomes discoloured.

- If you have a severe food allergy, contact the airline in advance, stating the type and severity of your allergy. If you are allergic to peanuts, ask whether the flight is peanut free (many airlines now ban peanuts).

- As soon as you arrive, locate the nearest telephone and find out the telephone numbers of the nearest doctor, ambulance service, and hospital accident and emergency department.

- Remember that the telephone number for the emergency services (999 in the UK) varies from country to country.

- Teach your travelling companions what to do if you have an acute severe allergic reaction.

- Take with you a letter from your doctor explaining what your medication is and confirming that it is for your own personal use. This should avoid any problems at Customs and Excise inspections.

- If you do not speak the language of the country that you are visiting, Allergy UK and the Anaphylaxis Campaign (see 'Useful information', page 133) can provide you with a range of cards carrying translations of important messages.

Bon voyage!

Finance

Having an allergic condition can be costly, not only because of all those prescription costs but also because of the cost of special diets, non-allergenic and protective bedding, and other special equipment that you might need.

If you are not exempt from paying prescription charges, a pre-payment certificate may reduce the cost. Currently, if you require more than five items in a four-month period, pre-payment works out cheaper, because, after paying the flat fee, all prescriptions are free, no matter how many you need.

To obtain a pre-payment certificate contact your local health authority or ask at your pharmacy. Some medications are cheaper to buy over the counter from your pharmacist than paying a prescription charge. Your pharmacist can advise you on this. He or she can also provide you with a leaflet called *Are you entitled to help with health costs?*

If you need a special diet, some foodstuffs can be prescribed by your GP. Most people on special diets receive no financial help, but your modified diet need not be expensive. Allergy UK and the Anaphylaxis Campaign (see 'Useful information', page 133) are good sources of information about special cookbooks. All of the major supermarkets provide 'free-from' lists which can be very helpful in identifying foods that are safe for you to eat (see 'Useful information', page 133).

KEY POINTS

- With the right information and support, your children's schools will be able to cope with all issues relating to their allergic conditions

- Even children with severe allergies should be able to join in most activities at school

- With careful forward planning, a holiday can be a very enjoyable experience even if you have severe allergies

- Before you go on holiday, make sure that you have adequate medical insurance and, for the EU, take your EHIC (see page 126)

- If you are not exempt from paying prescription charges, a pre-payment certificate may reduce your costs

The future

Allergic diseases are becoming more common, and at present doctors can only treat these conditions, not cure them. However, we are gaining new knowledge all the time, and new drugs are being found and important discoveries are being made every year. One new drug is a monoclonal anti-IgE antibody, which has been shown to give improved asthma control and reduce symptoms in patients with allergic rhinitis. It is currently being trialled in other allergic conditions including food allergy.

We have learned a great deal recently about the factors that increase our children's chances of developing allergic diseases, and the result of this is that we can now start to develop prevention methods. Some of these are very simple, for example, ensuring that babies and young children are NEVER exposed to tobacco smoke. Others are more complex, and include the avoidance of certain allergens in the maternal diet during pregnancy, in the household environment during pregnancy, and in the infant's early postnatal environment.

Unfortunately, recent programmes looking at the effect of reducing the exposure of babies to a number of different food allergens while still in the womb have not shown any benefits, and it is too early to be able to offer advice about other early life allergen avoidance to families. However, there are a large number of research projects being done and, if you are interested in taking part in this type of medical research, one of the large research charities such as Allergy UK may be able to put you in contact with a local research group.

Major advances have been made in learning about the genetics of allergy. Our genetic material is found on our chromosomes, which are made of DNA and carry our genes – the units of genetic material that determine the characteristics that we inherit from our parents.

Scientists are currently identifying the genes responsible for the development of different allergic conditions. Once these genes are known, it may be possible to develop new drugs designed specifically to target certain aspects of the disease. In the longer term, it may be possible to repair faulty genes and provide a cure.

Work is also going on to investigate the possibility of immunising against allergy. Although this seems a very attractive option, we do not know yet whether a vaccine would be effective and, just as importantly, whether it would be safe. A vaccine against cat allergy is currently being assessed.

While we are waiting for these dreams to become reality, we can still take advantage of the new drugs that have been developed over the past few years. The newer antihistamines are virtually non-sedating, more effective and have the advantage of a once-a-day dosage schedule. The leukotriene receptor antagonists are showing great promise for selected patients, who are very enthusiastic about these drugs as they are taken by mouth. Tacrolimus and pimecrolimus offer a new way to treat eczema.

Finally, as you learn more about what happens when you have an allergic reaction, what the trigger factors of your allergies are and how to avoid them, you will be able to manage your symptoms more effectively and so improve the quality of your life and the lives of your loved ones. I hope that this book has succeeded in helping you achieve that.

Useful information

Useful addresses
General
Action Against Allergy
PO Box 278
Twickenham, Middx. TW1 4QQ
Tel: 020 8892 2711
Fax: 020 8892 4950
Email: AAA@actionagainstallergy.freeserve.co.uk
Website: www.actionagainstallergy.co.uk

A support charity, providing information (including holiday and accommodation), suppliers' lists, newsletter advice on specialist referral. Send an SAE for information.

Action on Smoking and Health (ASH)
102 Clifton Street
London EC2A 4HW
Tel: 020 7739 5902
Fax: 020 7613 0531
Email: enquiries@ash.org.uk
Website: www.ash.org.uk

A national organisation with branches throughout the UK. Campaigns on anti-smoking policies offering free

information on website or for sale from HQ. Catalogue
on request.

Allerayde Ltd
Freepost NG2687, 1B Enterprise Park, Brunel Drive
Newark, Notts NG24 2DZ
Tel: 01636 613609
Fax: 01636 612161
Email: info@allerayde.co.uk
Website: www.AlleraydeDirect.co.uk

Distributor of dustproof bedding and other products
such as sleeping suits for children and adults. Mail order
only; catalogue on request.

AllergyFree Direct Ltd
Maer Down Road
Bude, Cornwall EX23 8NG
Tel/fax: 01288 356396
Email: comments@allergyfreedirect.com
Website: www.allergyfreedirect.com

Mail order specialist for foods free from wheat, gluten,
milk and eggs; vegan and vegetarian foods also
available. The website is easy to navigate with the
categories clearly labelled and giving the ingredients
used for each product. It also contains a glossary.

Allergy UK
(formerly British Allergy Foundation)
3 White Oak Square, London Road
Swanley, Kent BR8 7AG
Helpline: 01322 619898
Fax: 01322 663480

Email: info@allergyuk.org
Website: www.allergyuk.org

Encompasses all types of allergies, food and chemical sensitivities, and offers information, quarterly newsletter and support network; translation cards available for travel abroad £15. Annual subscription for 2005: £20.

Anaphylaxis Campaign
PO Box 275, Farnborough
Hampshire GU14 6SX
Tel: 01252 373793
Fax: 01252 377140
Helpline: 01252 542029
Email: info@anaphylaxis.org.uk
Website: www.anaphylaxis.org.uk

Campaigns for better awareness of life-threatening allergic reactions from food and other allergies to bee and wasp stings. Produces a wide range of educational news sheets and has extensive support network.

Asda
Customer Services Department, Asda House
Great Wilson Street
Leeds LS11 5AD
Tel: 0113 243 5435
Fax: 0113 241 8666
Helpline: 0500 100055
Minicom: 0800 068 3003
Website: www.asda.co.uk

'Free-from' booklets available on request and on website.

Asthma UK
Summit House, 70 Wilson Street
London EC2A 2DB
Tel: 020 7786 4900
Fax: 020 7256 6075
Helpline: 08457 010203
Email: asthmanurse.org.uk
Website: www.asthma.org.uk

Publications about asthma and its management and helpline run by team of asthma nurse specialists. Funds medical research and has local support groups.

Benefits Enquiry Line
Tel: 0800 882200
Website: www.dwp.gov.uk
Minicom: 0800 243355
N. Ireland: 0800 220674

Government agency giving information and advice on sickness and disability benefits for people with disabilities and their carers.

Boots Customer Services
1 Thane Road
Nottingham NG2 3AA
Tel: 0115 950 6111
Helpline: 0845 070 8090
Website: www.boots.com

Will provide, on request, 'free-from' lists on their own-brand products.

British Society for Allergy and Clinical Immunology (BSACI)
17 Doughty Street
London WC1N 2PL
Tel: 020 7404 0278
Fax: 020 7404 0280
Email: info@bsaci.org
Website: www.bsaci.org

Produces a regularly updated list of NHS allergy clinics throughout the country.

Coeliac UK
PO Box 220
High Wycombe, Bucks HP11 2HY
Tel: 01494 437278
Fax: 01494 474349
Helpline: 0870 444 8804
Email: admin@coeliac.co.uk
Website: www.coeliac.co.uk

Provides information and support for people medically diagnosed with coeliac disease or dermatitis herpetiformis.

Co-op
Customer Services, CWS Ltd
PO Box 53, New Century House
Manchester M60 4ES
Tel: 0161 834 1212
Helpline: 0800 068 6727
Minicom: 0800 068 4244
Email: customer.relations@co-op.co.uk
Website: www.co-op.co.uk

Will provide, on request, 'free-from' lists free of charge for their own-brand products.

Cosmetic Toiletry & Perfumery Association (CTPA) Ltd

Josaron House, 5–7 John Princes Street
London W1G 0JN
Tel: 020 7491 8891
Fax: 020 7493 8061
Email: info@ctpa.org.uk
Website: www.ctpa.org.uk

Association for professionals, providing details of cosmetic ingredients only to its members, not the general public.

Department for Education and Skills (DfES)

PO Box 5050, Sherwood Park
Annesley, Notts NG15 0DL
Helpline: 0870 000 2288
Publications: 0845 602 2260
Email: dfes@prolog.uk.com
Website: www.dfes.gov.uk

Government information centre that refers callers to different departments as appropriate.

Department for Environment, Food & Rural Affairs (DEFRA) (formerly MAFF)

Information Resource Centre, Nobel House
17 Smith Square, London SW1P 3JR
Helpline: 0845 933 5577
Email: helpline@defra.gsi.gov.uk
Website: www.defra.gov.uk

Implements Government policies and publishes information about environmental, rural and farming matters
and food production. Enquiries about allergies now
dealt with by the Food Standards Agency (see below).

Department of Health
PO Box 77
London SE1 6XH
Tel: 020 7210 4850
Fax: 01623 724524
Helpline: 0800 555777 (health literature line)
Textline: 01623 756236
Website: www.doh.gov.uk

Produces and distributes literature about public health.
Enquiries about allergies now dealt with by the Food
Standards Agency (see below). Website link 'Health
Advice for Travellers' gives details of how to apply
for an EHIC (supersedes form E111 – see page 126).
See also 'Useful publications (Travel)' on page 153.

Food Standards Agency
Aviation House, 125 Kingsway
London WC2B 6NH
Tel: 020 7276 8000
Publications: 0845 606 0667
Website: www.foodstandards.gov.uk

For queries about specific sensitivities or allergies:
Additives: 020 7276 8570
Allergies and intolerances: 020 7276 8533
Chemical safety: 020 7276 8522
Contaminants: 020 7276 8710
Novel foods: 020 7276 8596

Foresight
178 Hawthorn Road
West Bognor, West Sussex PO21 2UY
Tel: 01243 868001
Fax: 01243 868180
Website: www.foresight-preconception.org.uk

Gives advice and counselling on preconceptual care;
sells publications, vitamins and minerals.

Golden Key
1 Hare Street
Sheerness, Kent ME12 1AH
Tel: 01795 663403
Fax: 01795 661356

Provides engraving service for SOS identification
jewellery. Individual service available by mail order.

Health and Safety Executive
Information Services, Caerphilly Business Park
Caerphilly CF83 3GG
Helpline: 0845 345 0055 (8am–6pm Mon–Fri)
Textphone: 0845 408 9577
Fax: 0845 408 9566
Email: hseinfoline@natbrit.com
Website: www.hse.gov.uk

Offers information and advice about health and safety
regulations in the workplace and their implementation.

Holiday Care
7th Floor, Sunley House, 4 Bedford Park
Croydon CR0 2AP

Tel: 0845 124 9974
Fax: 0845 124 9972
Helpline: 0845 124 9971
Minicom: 0845 124 9976
Email: info@holidaycare.org
Website: www.holidaycare.org.uk

Provides holiday advice on venues and tour operators for people with special needs, including transport, insurance, oxygen supplies, etc. in the UK and abroad. Publishes information sheets on overseas destinations. Offers professional consultancy service to the tourism industry.

Institute of Translation and Interpreting
Fortuna House, South Fifth Street
Milton Keynes MK9 2EU
Tel: 01908 325250
Fax: 01908 325259
Email: info@iti.org.uk
Website: www.iti.org.uk

Institute for translators and interpreters; most languages covered.

Marks and Spencer
Customer Services, Chester Business Park
Wrexham Road
Chester CH4 9GA
Tel: 0845 302 1234
Fax: 0845 303 0170
Email: retailcustomer.services@marks-and-spencer.com
Website: www.marksandspencer.com

Will provide, on request, information on own-brand foods that are suitable for special diets (diabetes not included)

MedicAlert

1 Bridge Wharf, 156 Caledonian Road
London N1 9UU
Tel: 020 7833 3034
Fax: 020 7278 0647
Helpline: 0800 581420
Email: info@medicalert.org.uk
Website: www.medicalert.org.uk

Provides emergency identification with body-worn jewellery for people with hidden medical conditions and allergies. A 24-hour emergency telephone accepts reverse charge calls; can access personal details from anywhere in the world in over 100 languages.

Wm Morrison Supermarkets plc (previously Safeways)

Customer Service Department, Parry Lane
Bradford BD4 8TD
Tel: 01274 356000
Fax: 01274 356780
Website: www.morrisons.co.uk

Will provide, on request, information on own-brand products that are suitable for special diets.

National Eczema Society

Hill House, Highgate Hill
London N19 5NA
Tel: 020 7281 3553

Fax: 020 7281 6395
Helpline: 0870 241 3604 (Mon–Fri 8am–8pm;
textphone also on this number)
Website: www.eczema.org

Provides information, newsletter and helpline for
people with eczema and for parents of children with
eczema. Has local support network.

National Pollen Research Unit
University College Worcester, Henwick Grove
Worcester WR2 6AJ
Tel: 01905 855000
Email: pollen@worc.ac.uk
Website: www.worc.ac.uk

This website offers pollen forecasts and links to other
allergy-related organisations.

**National Institute for Health and Clinical
Excellence (NICE)**
MidCity Place, 71 High Holborn
London WC1V 6NA
Tel: 020 7067 5800
Fax: 020 7067 5801
Email: nice@nice.nhs.uk
Website: www.nice.org.uk

Provides national guidance on the promotion of good
health and the prevention and treatment of ill-health.
Patient information leaflets are available for each piece
of guidance issued.

Prodigy Website
Sowerby Centre for Health Informatics at Newcastle (SCHIN)
Bede House, All Saints Business Centre
Newcastle upon Tyne NE1 2ES
Tel: 0191 243 6100
Fax: 0191 243 6101
Email: prodigy-enquiries@schin.co.uk
Website: www.prodigy.nhs.uk/PILS/indexself.asp

A website mainly for GPs giving information for patients listed by disease plus named self-help organisations.

Safeways
See Wm Morrison Supermarkets.

Sainsbury's Supermarkets Ltd
Customer Services, 33 Holborn
London EC1N 2HT
Helpline: 0800 636262
Website: www.sainsbury.co.uk

'Free-from' lists for various special diets available on web and on request.

Somerfield Stores Ltd
Customer Services, Somerfield House, Whitchurch Lane
Bristol BS14 0TJ
Tel: 0117 935 9359
Helpline: 0117 935 6669
Website: www.somerfield.co.uk

'Free-from' lists for various special diets available on request.

SOS Talisman Ltd
Talman Ltd, 21 Grays Corner, Ley Street
Ilford, Essex IG2 7RQ
Tel: 020 8554 5579
Fax: 020 8554 1090
Website: www.sos-talisman.com

Produces a selection of identification jewellery available
by mail order and through branches of Boots the
Chemists. Medical details are supplied on folded pieces
of paper that are incorporated into various items of
jewellery.

Tesco
Customer Services, Freepost SCO2298, Baird Avenue
Dundee DD1 9NF
Helpline: 0800 505555
Fax: 01382 822230
Email: customer.service@tesco.co.uk
Website: www.tesco.com

'Free-from' lists for various special diets available on
request.

Waitrose
Nutritional Advice Centre, Waitrose,
Southern Industrial Area, Doncastle Road
Bracknell, Berks RG12 8YA
Tel: 01344 424680
Fax: 01344 824978
Helpline: 0800 188884
Nutritionist: 01344 824975
Email: customer_service@waitrose.co.uk
Website: www.waitrose.com

'Free-from' lists for various special diets available on request.

Complementary therapies
British Acupuncture Council
63 Jeddo Road
London W12 9HQ
Tel: 020 8735 0400
Fax: 020 8735 0404
Email: info@acupuncture.org.uk
Website: www.acupuncture.org.uk

Professional body offering lists of qualified acupuncture therapists. Can refer to accredited institutions for training.

British Homeopathic Association
Hahnemann House, 20 Park Street West
Luton LU1 3BE
Tel: 08704 443 950
Fax: 08704 443 960
Email: info@trusthomeopathy.org
Website: www.trusthomeopathy.org

Professional body offering lists of qualified homeopathic practitioners.

British Medical Acupuncture Society (BMAS)
BMAS House, 3 Winnington Court
Northwich, Cheshire CW8 1AQ
Tel: 01606 786782
Fax: 01606 786783
Email: admin@medical-acupuncture.org.uk
Website: www.medical-acupuncture.co.uk

Professional body offering training in acupuncture to registered health-care professionals and lists of accredited practitioners in local areas.

General Chiropractic Council
44 Wicklow Street
London WC1X 9HL
Tel: 020 7713 5155
Fax: 020 7713 5844
Helpline: 0845 601 1796
Email: enquiries@gcc-uk.org
Website: www.gcc-uk.org

Professional body for chiropractors that can provide details of registered practitioners in your area.

General Osteopathic Council
Osteopathy House, 176 Tower Bridge Road
London SE1 3LU
Tel: 020 7357 6655
Fax: 020 7357 0011
Email: info@osteopathy.org.uk
Website: www.osteopathy.org.uk

Regulatory body that offers information about osteopathy to the public and lists of accredited osteopaths in local areas.

Institute of Complementary Medicine
PO Box 194
London SE16 7QZ
Tel: 020 7237 5165
Fax: 020 7237 5175
Email: info@i-c-m.org.uk
Website: www.i-c-m.org.uk

A registered charity formed as an umbrella for complementary medicine groups. Recommends approved training courses and has register of accredited British practitioners. For information please send SAE with two first-class stamps.

International Federation of Reflexologists
76–78 Edridge Road
Croydon, Surrey CR0 1EF
Tel: 020 8645 9134
Fax: 020 8649 9291
Email: info@IntFedReflexologists.org
Website: www.intfedreflexologists.org

Professional body representing reflexologists internationally, offering information to the public and advice on suitable training.

National Institute of Medical Herbalists
Elm House, 54 Mary Arches Street
Exeter EX4 3BA
Tel: 01392 426022
Fax: 01392 498963
Email: nimh@ukexeter.freeserve.co.uk
Website: www.NIMH.org.uk

Professional body representing qualified, practising medical herbalists. Offers list of accredited medical herbalists in your area. Please send an SAE.

Register of Chinese Herbal Medicine
Office 5, Ferndale Business Centre, 1 Exeter Street
Norwich NR2 4QB
Tel: 01603 623994

Fax: 01603 667557
Email: herbmed@rchm.co.uk
Website: www.rchm.co.uk

Regulatory body holding register of practitioners in the UK appropriately trained in Chinese herbal medicine. For list of qualified members, an SAE is requested.

Medical equipment
Clement Clarke International Ltd
Edinburgh Way
Harlow, Essex CM20 2TT
Tel: 01279 414969
Fax: 01279 456304
Email: resp@clement-clarke.com
Website: www.clement-clarke.com

Suppliers of peak flowmeters, spacers and nebulisers.

Dunlopillo & Slumberland
Salmon Fields, Ryton
Oldham OL2 6SB
Tel: 0161 628 2565
Fax: 0161 628 4820
Email: enquiries@dunlopillo.co.uk
Website: www.dunlopillo.co.uk

Manufacturers of latex foam mattresses, pillows and beds.

Medivac Healthcare Ltd
Freepost LON12778
London NW11 6YR
Tel: 0845 130 6969
Fax: 0845 130 6868

Helpline: 0845 130 6164
Email: medivacuk@aol.com
Website: www.medivac.co.uk

Supplies specialised vacuum cleaners, bedding, air filters, etc. for those with asthma, eczema, rhinitis, etc.

Profile Therapeutics plc (formerly Medic-Aid Ltd)
Heath Place
Bognor Regis, West Sussex PO22 9SL
Tel: 0870 770 3434
Fax: 0870 770 3433
Email: info@profiletherapeutics.com
Website: www.profilehs.com

Supplies nebulisers, compressors, facemasks and spacer devices.

Vitalograph Ltd
Maids Moreton House, Maids Moreton
Buckingham MK18 1SW
Tel: 01280 827110
Fax: 01280 823302
Email: sales@vitalograph.co.uk
Website: www.vitalograph.co.uk

Supplies spirometers and emergency resuscitation equipment as well as training on their use.

VK Direct (previously Vorwerk (UK) Ltd)
Maxon House, Hogwood Lane
Finchampstead, Berks RG40 4QW
Tel: 0118 973 8040
Fax: 0118 973 5014

Website: www.VKdirect.co.uk
Service Department: 0844 800 0123

Suppliers of vacuum cleaners.

Further websites
www.allallergy.net
Big website giving list of allergy-related websites.

www.allergies.about.com
All about allergies, in user-friendly language.

www.allerex.ca
All about how to use the EpiPen.

www.amazon.com
On-line bookshop.

www.boots.com
Information on products including those for allergy.

www.foodallergy.org
Website of the Food Allergy and Anaphylaxis Network
(a non-profit-making organisation in the USA).

www.peanutallergy.com
American site on peanut allergy.

Useful publications
In addition to the publications listed here, the various
allergy associations, organisations and self-help groups
publish a wide range of magazines, booklets, leaflets
and fact sheets. Contact them at the addresses given
for an up-to-date publications list.

General
Joanne Clough (1998) *Allergies at Your Fingertips*. London: Class Publishing.

Myron Lipkowitz (1994) *Allergies A–Z*. Facts on File.

Anne Woodham (1994) *HEA Guide to Complementary Medicine and Therapies*. London: Health Education Authority.

M. Eric Gershwin (1992) *Living Allergy Free*. London: Humana Press.

Asthma
Mark Levy, Sean Hilton and Greta Barnes (1997) *Asthma at Your Fingertips*, 2nd edn. London: Class Publishing.

Jenny Lewis with the National Asthma Campaign (1996) *The Asthma Handbook*. London: Vermilion.

John Donaldson (1994) *Living with Asthma and Hayfever*, revised edn. Harmondsworth: Penguin.

If you have asthma because of your work, NI237, issued by the Department of Social Security and available on request from your local Social Security offices, may be helpful.

Skin allergies
David J. Atherton (1995) *Eczema in Childhood – the Facts*, revised edn. Oxford: Oxford University Press.

Jenny Lewis with the National Eczema Society (1994) *The Eczema Handbook*. London: Vermilion.

Hay fever
Deryk Williams, Anna Williams and Laura Croker
(1997) *Living with Asthma and Hayfever*. London:
Piatkus Books.

Education
Your Guide to the NHS (formerly the Patient's Charter),
published by the Department of Health (single copies
available free of charge by calling 0800 555777).

Special Educational Needs – A guide for parents,
published by the Department for Education and Skills
(single copies available free from the DfES Publications
Centre by calling 0845 602 2260).

Supporting Pupils with Medical Needs in Schools,
published by the Department for Education and Skills
(single copies available free from the DfES Publications
Centre by calling 0845 602 2260).

Travel
Health Advice for Travellers, published by the
Department of Health (single copies available free of
charge by calling 0800 555777). Also contains details
of how to apply for an EHIC (see page 126).

The internet as a source of further information

After reading this book, you may feel that you would
like further information on the subject. The internet is
of course an excellent place to look and there are many
websites with useful information about medical
disorders, related charities and support groups.

It should always be remembered, however, that the internet is unregulated and anyone is free to set up a website and add information to it. Many websites offer impartial advice and information that has been compiled and checked by qualified medical professionals. Some, on the other hand, are run by commercial organisations with the purpose of promoting their own products. Others still are run by pressure groups, some of which will provide carefully assessed and accurate information whereas others may be suggesting medications or treatments that are not supported by the medical and scientific community.

Unless you know the address of the website you want to visit – for example, www.familydoctor.co.uk – you may find the following guidelines useful when searching the internet for information.

Search engines and other searchable sites

Google (www.google.co.uk) is the most popular search engine used in the UK, followed by Yahoo! (http://uk. yahoo.com) and MSN (www.msn.co.uk). Also popular are the search engines provided by Internet Service Providers such as Tiscali and other sites such as the BBC site (www.bbc.co.uk).

In addition to the search engines that index the whole web, there are also medical sites with search facilities, which act almost like mini-search engines, but cover only medical topics or even a particular area of medicine. Again, it is wise to look at who is responsible for compiling the information offered to ensure that it is impartial and medically accurate. The NHS Direct site (www.nhsdirect.nhs.uk) is an example of a searchable medical site.

Links to many British medical charities can be found at the Association of Medical Research Charities' website (www.amrc.org.uk) and at Charity Choice (www. charitychoice.co.uk).

Search phrases

Be specific when entering a search phrase. Searching for information on 'cancer' will return results for many different types of cancer as well as on cancer in general. You may even find sites offering astrological information. More useful results will be returned by using search phrases such as 'lung cancer' and 'treatments for lung cancer'. Both Google and Yahoo! offer an advanced search option that includes the ability to search for the exact phrase; enclosing the search phrase in quotes, that is, 'treatments for lung cancer', will have the same effect. Limiting a search to an exact phrase reduces the number of results returned but it is best to refine a search to an exact match only if you are not getting useful results with a normal search. Adding 'UK' to your search term will bring up mainly British sites, so a good phrase might be 'lung cancer' UK (don't include UK within the quotes).

Always remember the internet is international and unregulated. It holds a wealth of valuable information but individual sites may be biased, out of date or just plain wrong. Family Doctor Publications accepts no responsibility for the content of links published in this series.

Index

Your pages

We have included the following pages because they may help you manage your illness or condition and its treatment.

Before an appointment with a health professional, it can be useful to write down a short list of questions of things that you do not understand, so that you can make sure that you do not forget anything.

Some of the sections may not be relevant to your circumstances.

We are always pleased to receive constructive criticism or suggestions about how to improve the books. You can contact us at:

Email: familydoctor@btinternet.com
Letter: Family Doctor Publications
         PO Box 4664
         Poole
         BH15 1NN

Thank you

Health-care contact details

Name:

Job title:

Place of work:

Tel:

Name:

Job title:

Place of work:

Tel:

Name:

Job title:

Place of work:

Tel:

Name:

Job title:

Place of work:

Tel:

Significant past health events – illnesses/operations/investigations/treatments

Event	Month	Year	Age (at time)

Appointments for health care

Name:

Place:

Date:

Time:

Tel:

Name:

Place:

Date:

Time:

Tel:

Name:

Place:

Date:

Time:

Tel:

Name:

Place:

Date:

Time:

Tel:

Appointments for health care

Name:

Place:

Date:

Time:

Tel:

Name:

Place:

Date:

Time:

Tel:

Name:

Place:

Date:

Time:

Tel:

Name:

Place:

Date:

Time:

Tel:

Current medication(s) prescribed by your doctor

Medicine name:

Purpose:

Frequency & dose:

Start date:

End date:

Medicine name:

Purpose:

Frequency & dose:

Start date:

End date:

Medicine name:

Purpose:

Frequency & dose:

Start date:

End date:

Medicine name:

Purpose:

Frequency & dose:

Start date:

End date:

Other medicines/supplements you are taking, not prescribed by your doctor

Medicine/treatment:

Purpose:

Frequency & dose:

Start date:

End date:

Medicine/treatment:

Purpose:

Frequency & dose:

Start date:

End date:

Medicine/treatment:

Purpose:

Frequency & dose:

Start date:

End date:

Medicine/treatment:

Purpose:

Frequency & dose:

Start date:

End date:

Questions to ask at appointments
(Note: do bear in mind that doctors work under great time pressure, so long lists may not be helpful for either of you)